REIMAGINING MIDLIFE

WOMEN WHO REINVENTED THEMSELVES FOR THEIR SECOND ACT

Mary Eisenhauer

Midlife Reinvention: Lessons for the Next Half

Copyright 2024: Mary Eisenhauer
All rights reserved. No part of this book may be reproduced, excerpted, digitized, stored or used in any form except by a reviewer quoting brief passages allowed under fair use.

Cover image: Depositphotos.com

For the residents of 34 Meadowood, past and present;
the loves of my life.

For Mom and Dad, for summer reading programs,
weekend writing workshops, and my liberal arts education.

For Grammy, for assuring me I could do anything
I set my mind to.

Contents

Foreword 9

Back to School 11
- Tyra Hatcher 13
- Karen Juliano 21
- Amanda Mowbray 29
- Lori Reichel 35
- Sherry Rigel 41

Business Women 47
- Kavita Ahuja 49
- Marie Ambusk 55
- Kimchi Chow 61
- Marie Gettel-Gilmartin 67
- Tracy Vontélle Green and Nancey Flowers Harris 73

Healing and Helping 83
- Jackie Capers Brown 85
- Chantal Coupal 95
- Jennifer Faretra 101
- Gael Hogan 107
- Ellen Kaye 113
- Veronica Robles 119

Passion Projects 127
- Carline Bengtsson 129
- Sandy DeWeese 135
- Melissa Jenkins Mangili 141
- Andrea Koehler 149
- Kyoko Nagano 155
- Deborah Peel 161
- Monica Stellmacher 167

(more)

Contents *(continued)*

Relocation and Travel 175
  Harumi Gondo 177
  Lisa LaHiff 183
  Lyliana Morales 193
  Joanne Robb 201

Serial Reinvention 209
  Molly Barker 211
  Ann Bordeleau 219
  Becky McCord 225

You're More Than You Knew 231
  Lorraine Connell 233
  Kendra Hackett 239
  Sue Loncaric 247
  JoAna McCoy 253
  Katie O'Leary 259

Maps for My Own Journey 265

About the Author 267

Foreword

The year leading up to my 50th birthday was full of dread and apprehension. Fifty was halfway through middle age, the beginning of a downward slide. Society tends to put women in boxes as they age. Wives. Mothers. Grandmothers. Caretakers. Fashion options start to dwindle. Ageism in the workplace becomes more prevalent. Menopause strikes, accompanied by confusion and frustration. Once we hit our 40s, and certainly the age of 50, we're instantly less interesting and less attractive, and therefore less valuable. None of this sat well with me. Surely, midlife couldn't be that bleak.

Turning 50 brought conversations with my friends and co-workers. Many of us were finished with or closing in on the end of raising children. Many of us had worked in the same careers for decades, careers that no longer provided the fulfillment they once did. Our parents were aging or had passed away. We were married, remarried, single, or questioning our choices. Most of us were saying, "What now?" Something about hitting midlife forced a moment of truth for us. We knew we wanted different things for ourselves, but was 'different' actually possible?

On a random winter day in 2022, a conversation with an acquaintance forced my own moment of truth. This woman was re-entering the workforce after years of staying home with her children. We discussed the challenges of marketing her skills after more than a decade of unpaid work, and of reinventing herself at this stage of life. This conversation sent me down a path of finding women in midlife who had reinvented themselves: women who decided during in their mid-40s, 50s, or early 60s to make bold decisions about the way they would live their lives. They were thinking about making career transitions, starting businesses, taking on passion projects, traveling, or initiating lifestyle changes.

The year that I spent interviewing women for this book will sit in my memory as one of the best of my life. What started as a project based on American women ultimately extended across the world. Meeting women from all backgrounds, from all over the world, and learning about their challenges and transformations has been truly life-affirming. Whether through necessity or desire, these women have boldly reinvented themselves during a time in life when society tells them their value has diminished.

These women are badass, resilient, determined, and cool. They're beautiful, smart, and no-nonsense. And, now, they feel like friends. Coming out of the long, grim years of the pandemic, I can't think of a better way to spend free time than connecting with these women and telling their stories.

~ Mary Eisenhauer, 2024

Back to School

Higher education can provide professional opportunities. Degrees tend to open doors to compensation, health benefits, and increasingly responsible professional roles. In tight job markets, degrees differentiate job candidates.

But beyond financial and professional rewards, higher education impacts a person's mental and emotional health. A degree represents a sense of control—it's something that cannot be taken away.

A degree can also be a path to reinvention in midlife. The women in this section pursued studies in fields they became passionate about during their decades of professional and life experience.

Tyra Hatcher

Give Yourself Permission

Tyra has always followed her passions, embracing education, gardening, and hiking with confidence, allowing her interests to give her joy. She says it's all about learning to give yourself permission to do what you want. Now a real estate broker, she lives outside of Portland, Maine.

Tyra Hatcher learned early that role models aren't always positive influences.

"Growing up, all the women in my family just worked themselves to death. They worked, and they took care of family, and they volunteered, and they did stuff at church and for their friends. If you were not exhausted at the end of every day, you did not fulfill your goal in life."

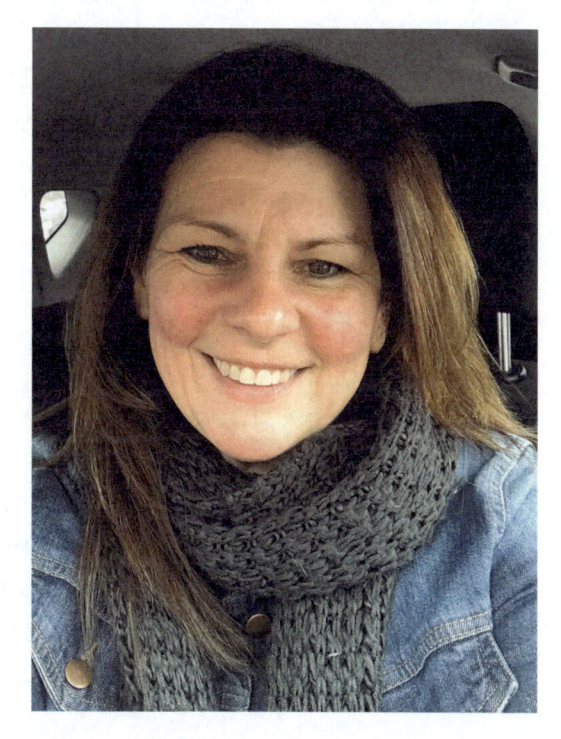

Later, she encountered, totally by accident, another kind of role model when she met a woman named Barbara through her local Buy Nothing group. When Tyra arrived to pick up chairs that Barbara had offered, she was also introduced to Barbara's Icelandic horses. "I touched the first one and I started to cry, like uncontrollable sobbing, crying for 20 minutes. I couldn't stop. I just I just kept looking over at Barbara to say, 'I'm so sorry; I don't know why I'm crying.' Barbara warmly responded, 'Sometimes they do that to you'."

Tyra's new friend was also a sailing captain. "She's just done so many interesting things in her life—just whatever she wanted to do. I left that day feeling that, when you give yourself space and you follow your curiosity and your instincts, you never know where it's going to take you. When you let that happen, how beautiful it is. It's changed my life."

Tyra says she's been forced by life circumstances to reinvent herself several times. Now, in mid-life, "I've gotten to a point where making money and doing what other people expect of me is not as important as what I really care about, what I want, and what sits in my soul and aligns with what I believe a higher purpose is... I have given myself permission to be patient with myself, and gentle, and stop doing things all the time and just let things go."

On the floor, looking up

Tyra was born in Maine and completed her undergraduate degree in sociology at Wheaton College in Massachusetts.

After college, she spent five years in Thailand, her first husband's home country, and her first child was born there. Tyra embraced the Thai culture and the wonderful people around her and found work teaching English as a Foreign Language. Later, she became director of a branch of the language center where she taught.

Returning to Maine in 2002, Tyra took a chance and enrolled in a real estate course. "I had no idea if I would be successful selling real estate, but I followed my instinct and loved it."

When she and her husband divorced, she poured herself into her career. She remarried twice. Following her third husband's career, she moved to D.C. to study Portuguese before moving first to Brazil, then to Guyana, where she worked as the Community Liaison Coordinator for the U.S. State Department at the American Embassy.

By 2017, Tyra was back in Maine and she transitioned into her career selling real estate. But another divorce forced her into a period of reflection.

Tyra says she was distraught when she and her third husband separated in 2018. "When you get to the place that you are on the floor, looking up, there's nowhere else to go but up, right?" she says now. "Reinventing myself wasn't exactly because I wanted to. It was what was necessary. And I didn't feel up for the challenge in the beginning."

But she came to understand that she had to rely on herself. "It's going to be hard. Whether you are in a typical family and well-supported by your mother and father and family who love and cherish you, or you have nobody, you're still going to face death and disease and hardship, and you're going to have to walk it alone. And so, for me, it's in the loneliest space that I have found the most personal growth. It's been understanding that no one's coming to save me. No one's going to fix me. No one can do this for me. I'm the one who has to do it."

She needed to earn money but felt stuck in real estate. "I remember thinking, "Well, what's the rest of my life going to look like?"

"For the first time in my whole life, I wasn't responsible for anyone else," she says. Her children were grown and on their own. Even as a child, she'd been responsible for her younger brother while her parents worked. "Now, I was free to do whatever I wanted."

A conversation with her daughter prompted Tyra to write a list of goals. She had lost all the real estate she had in her second divorce, so she wanted to own a rental property. She wanted to travel more and be more physically fit. And she wanted to go back to school. A healthy list of goals, and Tyra's reinvention began.

The world outside

Tyra started hiking, in part to give herself space from turmoil at home. "I started hiking to physically and mentally remove myself from the conflicts." She started with short trail walks, learning to enjoy her own company.

Then a friend told her about The 4,000 Footers (sometimes called the NH48). New Hampshire has 48 mountain peaks higher than 4,000 feet in elevation, including Mount Washington, the tallest peak in the state and famous for having the world's strongest wind gusts, sometimes in excess of 200 miles per hour. Tyra's goal is to hike them all. "The more physically fit that I became and the more time I had out in the woods, the more I could think about my life goals, about what I wanted and how I was going to do it, and thinking of a different way to do it than maybe other people have done it. For me, transition has been dropping all my expectations around what I'm supposed to do and coming up with my own version of how I'm going to do my life—and then deciding along the way if I even want to keep doing it... I feel like this time in our life is like a zigzag."

She revisited the passion for gardening she'd found in 2006 when her son was ill and she was home taking care of him. "I started planting seeds and getting interested in gardening: watching the garden grow, recognizing the accomplishment,

Mary Eisenhauer

"I have given myself permission to be patient with myself, and gentle, and stop doing things all the time and just let things go."

and then being able to eat the fruits of my labor. It feels like, "I can take care of myself, and I can be resilient."

She became a certified Master Gardener in 2018 and has learned about food preservation, volunteering her time to talk about food insecurity.

Back to college

Tyra decided to go to graduate school for a degree in education, planning to work in college-level student affairs.

Tyra says the application process was interesting "because I had gotten to the point where I didn't have a lot of self-esteem." But she cried when she read the glowing recommendations written by her former teachers and colleagues and realized "I am a smart, accomplished woman who has worked really hard and achieved success. As a real estate agent, I've been a big part of other people's lives. I've helped people get through divorces and deaths in their families and transitions. And I have not been giving myself credit for any of the things I had been doing."

She worked very hard to get up to speed again. "I hadn't written anything longer than an e-mail in 25 years, and that first paper I wrote—I worked really hard on it and spent a lot of time on it. And I remember that there was a lot of joy in learning new things."

Tyra spent two years in graduate school, "just loving the process of learning something new, of being able to articulate my ideas to grow with the people in my class."

At almost 50, Tyra was older than many of the traditional students who had just completed their undergraduate studies. "Their experience was so different from mine, and in the beginning, I felt like that was a weakness or a separation. But what I quickly learned was that it was actually a strength because I had experience that they didn't have."

Tyra says grad school was hard and expensive, but says it was "really the first investment in myself."

A pandemic pivot

Tyra completed her graduate degree in 2020—just in time for COVID-19 lockdowns to prevent her from pursuing her new career. But she was still determined to work with students. Her solution was to teach classes for real estate agents.

"I feel like there are people who might say, 'Oh, you didn't do anything with your degree,' but I absolutely did. That changed me as a person, changed me as a human being. Being able to teach brought me to a place of rebuilding my confidence, of reassessing my life goals."

Many choices

Tyra says "I used to have a lot of anxiety about not knowing what I wanted to do with my life, and now I realize I don't have to do just one thing... Now I want to be a few different things. I want to be a real estate agent. I love being part of people's stories. I love selling houses. And I want to be a gardener and help other people do that because there's a lot of joy and beauty in being outside and getting your hands in the dirt."

Tyra says the biggest challenge of being self-employed is feeling that every hour has to produce income, that, "...if I'm not working, not producing money, my time is not valuable—instead of understanding that the downtime that I take for myself makes me a more productive, happier person." She has finally learned to prioritize what she needs and wants. "I no longer feel like I need to explain to other people, which means I don't need to explain to myself... Now, I'm really able to stand in my own space, be proud of what I do, and let the rest just work itself out."

She has reinvigorated her real estate business by focusing on distressed properties, working with first-time home buyers and sellers facing foreclosure.

Finding the flow

"The most important relationship has to be with yourself, and I never investigated or invested time in that," Tyra says. She says part of the process is becoming comfortable with your own thoughts, "even sadness or thoughts or feelings that people feel are negative. They're not negative, they're just feelings.

"When you get comfortable with being lonely or alone, you become practiced in it. And when you become practiced in anything, you become more comfortable and more capable. That's like the grad school piece: it wasn't that I wasn't a good writer. It's that I wasn't practiced in writing. As I became practiced in writing, I became more confident. And as I became more confident, my writing became better because it started to flow.

"Midlife is flow. We have been resisting or fighting or pushing or dragging people and things in jobs and ideas behind us for so long, that when you get to the place where you just drop it all and let it be, it's quite amazing."

Tyra doesn't waste time on regrets. "I don't play that game anymore because I can't go back. I'm not going to put any energy into it. And I wouldn't want to go back. Even in the worst, darkest days of my life, there are things that have come into my life that are beautiful. If I won the lottery today and my life changed forever, what would I do differently? For the most part, I wouldn't do anything differently. I would still be gardening, and sending postcards to friends, and selling real estate to people I like working with, and thinking about the next adventure I want to be on."

Karen Juliano

The "Big Five-O"

Turning 50 triggered an identity crisis for Karen, but she turned it into a journey of self-discovery that has taken her away from corporate jobs and towards writing and leadership. Karen divides her time between Maine and Florida.

The "Big Five-O" forced Karen Juliano to make some big changes.

"I felt like I didn't have a passion, that I didn't have this brass ring that I was going for. I had been searching for my creative outlet. I have had this ongoing romance with thinking that I wanted to be a writer, wanting to write and have that kind of creativity in any way. I have decided to do that."

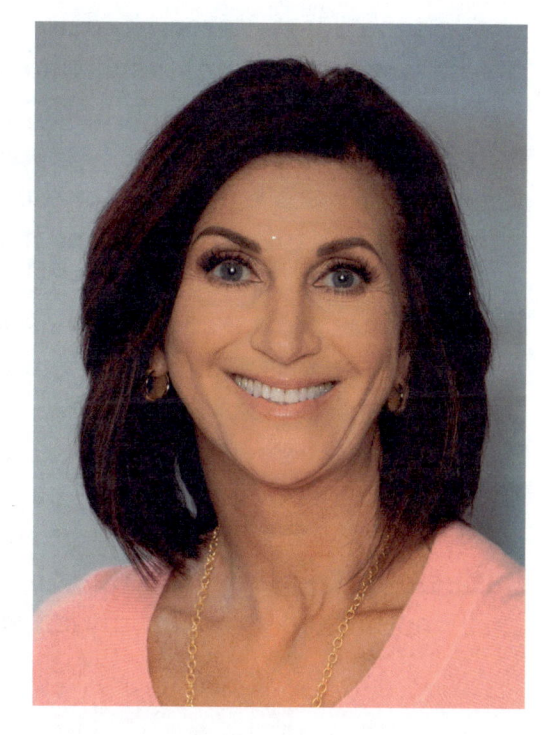

"I think it was just mainly coming from a place at this stage of my life where I have no desire for any drudgery at all. There's no room in this half of my life for something that I do not feel completely."

Building a business

Karen is not afraid of hard work. She bought a specialty retail store when she was 24, and over the next 16 years, she was self-employed as she built and expanded it. "It was challenging financially," she says, "but I did it, and after six years I had more than doubled the size of my store. And I was known throughout the city for having creative window displays. I made a point to create beautiful, unique displays and people came from all over the city to see them. At the time I didn't realize what a significant creative outlet this was for me, and how important creativity would be in my life."

During that time, she married and had two children, but the relationship deteriorated as she and her husband spent considerable time apart. Karen needed validation from her husband, but he was neither emotionally nor physically available to give it. They ended up divorcing, with Karen taking on the majority of parenting. She felt she had stepped onto a hamster wheel as her days consisted of caring for the kids, driving them to extracurricular activities, and running her business. Little else.

Life became increasingly difficult as her parents and a couple of siblings passed away in quick succession. Between her divorce and the loss of multiple family members, Karen's passion for her business fizzled and she lost the motivation to run it.

She then turned 40. She sold her business in 2010, just as the Great Recession was ending and the economy had tanked. Jobs were scarce. "I had essentially spent 16 years owning a business and putting everything I had into it. I sold it with virtually nothing to show for myself and that was a hard blow to my ego and self-esteem. What was my value if I didn't have my business?"

Because she had sold her business instead of filing for bankruptcy, she wasn't eligible for unemployment in the state of Maine. "I drained every cent I had to my name to be sure I made good on all of the commitments to my customers. I made sure that they had their merchandise, and I was left with nothing. It was my choice to do that—I needed to be done with that chapter of my life."

"Life kept kicking me when I was down. I got a divorce. I had challenges with my kids. My parents and a couple of siblings passed away. And I lost my business. " But Karen believes that "you're not handed any challenge or lesson that you can't handle. And I guess God, or the universe, or whoever, was giving me the proverbial knock upside the head for the majority of my life. And I finally got it. It was going to be hard but I needed to figure out a new direction for my life, something that was going to be meaningful."

The search for meaningful work

Her next professional venture was to manage the turnaround of a wholesale produce company. "I was responsible for the financial strength of the wholesale produce company. I moved on from there once I had overhauled the financial processes, and joined a major food company as a salesperson. It was this role where my earning potential really elevated.

"I was a month ahead on my mortgage. It was like a whole new world for me. I felt powerful. I felt strong. I wasn't scared anymore." And she continued to juggle her work and home lives. Her children were in high school and college, and her new financial status was well-timed. She could provide more for them with this new salary.

When she was recruited by a large payment processing

> "There are a lot of things that are involved in a reinvention. It isn't just a vocation."

company, Karen made the leap to supervise a small group in operations. "I took the 'grass is greener on the other side of the fence' approach," she says, lured by the stable hours. Her previous job was "24/7, weekends, everything," and the new position was "that quintessential 9 to 5." She reasoned with herself that she would be able to do both in this new job: provide for her children and spend precious time left with them as they became adults.

"But I hated it the moment I walked in there and saw my placard on a cubicle. I knew I'd made a mistake." The 'cube farm' she had signed on for was cold and uninviting, a place where her gender would hold her back and she couldn't trust her colleagues.

Karen found herself asking the same questions she'd faced after she sold her business. "It kind of became like another journey of, "How did I get here? Now I'm 45 and I'm trying to figure out again who I want to be when I grow up."

As the job crushed her spirit and her teenage daughter began to struggle, she decided to move on. She needed time and flexibility to support her daughter through major challenges, and to focus on what she wanted for herself. She took a series of small jobs to stay afloat.

Finding reinvention

In 2017 she learned about professional coach training. Being a coach could enable her to support and challenge others in attaining their personal and professional goals. "That was a pivotal point in my own self-awareness and development." Navigating her daughter's issues " catapulted me into a whole other stratosphere of personal work; and because of that, my relationship to other people, my relationship to myself, and how I look at personal growth and development." She set out on a path to fully understand her past, her mistakes, and her role in past conflicts. Reconciling her past would position her to coach others toward their own goals.

Karen believes the process of reconciling her past is more than just reading books or watching videos. "It's different. Really purposeful, intentional awareness, constructive introspection, and work on, 'How did I end up where I am today? What do I want to do with myself?'." She read many books, followed several self-help experts, and focused on making changes within herself to improve relationships with family and friends. In some cases, this meant drastically changing those relationships or even exiting them.

Karen once thought she wanted to climb the corporate ladder, but as her emotional intelligence grew, she couldn't imagine herself back in that world.

"I am choosing to be selective about where and with whom I invest myself and my time. Unfortunately, my last experience in a corporate environment demonstrated the need for more dynamic leadership. The toxicity was far too pervasive for me and left me feeling like working on those environments rather than in them better suits me."

This change in emotional intelligence pushed her to become certified as a coach. She completed a program and soon opened her own office for clients. This provided her with the flexibility and fulfillment she had been seeking.

The value of having a coach

As a coach herself, Karen understood the value of coaching, so she enlisted the help of not one, but two coaches. "You would think I could coach the hell out of myself. It just goes to show, though: no matter what we do, we still have obstacles within ourselves to overcome As women, we need external sources to either catapult us or reinforce us into what we already know and believe."

Working with coaches herself was a turning point. "It was very organic and authentic when I was asked the question: if I could do one thing and know that I wouldn't fail, what would I do? And without missing a beat, I said, 'I would write and publish a book'."

A writer's life

Karen enjoys writing short fiction but, although she has an intriguing life story, she has no urge to write a memoir. "I might sneak it into a fictitious character," she says. "Maybe I'll come to a place, at a certain point in time, to tell that story. I think it's a story worth telling because I know a lot of other parents have dealt with what I went through with my daughter. I'm just not there yet."

She finished her bachelor's degree in organizational leadership, but no longer had a passion for the field. She dedicated the months after graduation to seeing "where it leads, what kind of inspiration I have, how easily it flows–and then whether or not I go forward with pursuing the master's degree or not."

Still, she came to see her degree as validation, something she has craved throughout her life. "There's that gremlin inside me that's still seeking a level of credibility. Like, give me a spattering of letters after my name and then I'm legit."

But Karen says, "There are a lot of things that are involved in a reinvention. It isn't just a vocation." She calls her reinvention as a writer her "epiphany." "I'm hoping that, in the writing, I'll find that freedom. I'm hoping my soul will be freed, instead of feeling like I need all this external validation. I see writing as an opportunity to potentially experience that.

"My passion for writing fits what I want my life to look like. The life of a writer with a degree of solitude and the opportunity to be creative is what I want for this next phase of my life."

Karen has found her 50s to be freeing. "I don't feel compelled to just force my round peg into a square hole. I can say, 'No, I'm not doing that. That's not right for me.' It's liberating."

A transformative year

Karen's educational goals and writing aspirations have come together, at last. She began a master's degree in organizational leadership in January 2023 and completed it in December of the same year. The year was transformative. "It was an intense year and further solidified my journey of self-expansion. I discovered a renewed passion for leadership, emphasizing mental well-being in the workplace. I enjoy 'doing my work' and would really like to bring this concept to a working environment.

"The goal is for this to trickle down to children by making adults more knowledgeable about mental well-being, more emotionally intelligent, and able to see the value in integrating mental well-being practices in schools–and, therefore, gain their support for those initiatives."

Since then, she's been taking a much-needed break from intense schooling. "I have been traveling and writing. I will complete two short stories by adding illustrations to one story and a journal accompaniment to the other. The latter will hopefully inspire others to engage in their own personal 'work' and begin a journey of healing, growth, and joy, paving the way to greater personal and professional fulfillment." And perhaps these stories will be a new, improved type of validation for Karen.

Amanda Mowbray

Prioritizing A New Dream

Amanda used her return to college to propel herself out of a dead-end job and into a career in social work. Along the way, she became an avid runner and eventually an ultramarathoner. She has learned a lot about overcoming obstacles and following her dreams. Amanda lives in Virginia.

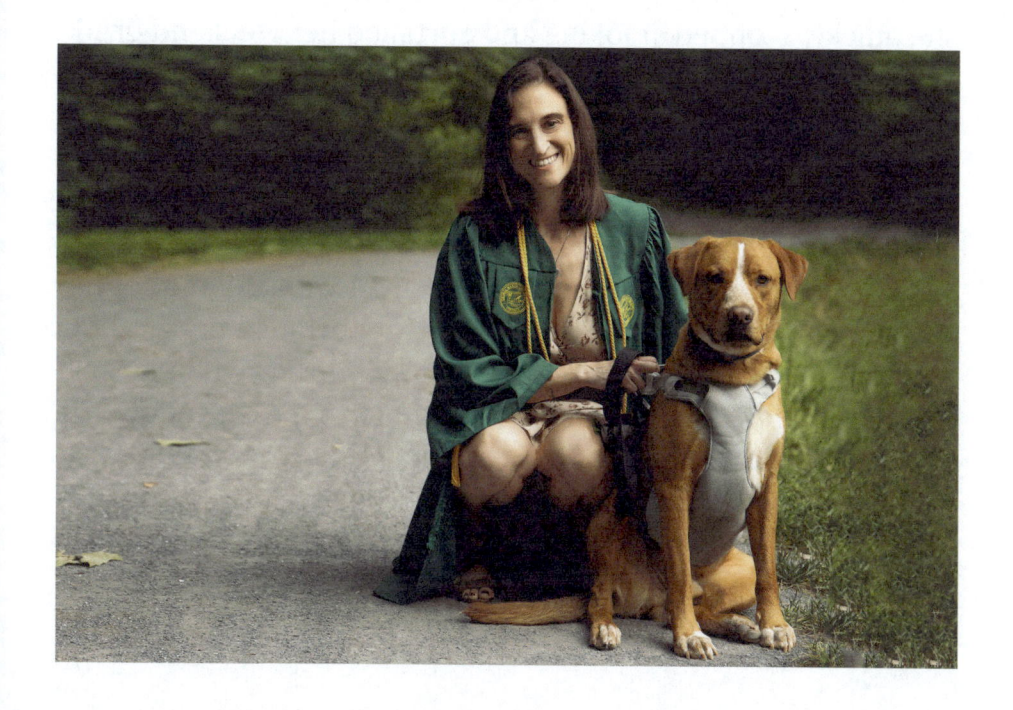

Amanda Mowbray knows a lot about persistence. She finished her associate degree when she was in her 20s, but never transferred to West Virginia University to do a four-year degree. "I decided I was going to go to WVU, then decided not to. I just sort of fell into things."

She worked in a series of jobs in the health insurance industry, from customer service to claims examiner. "Health insurance. Rarely anybody ever picks it as a career path," Amanda says. Nor was her personal life based on intentional choices. "I fell into a life of partying and hanging out, and I smoked and gained a lot of weight."

Her first reinvention

Amanda's wake-up call came when her father was diagnosed with congestive heart failure. His doctor convinced him that, if he quit smoking and drinking, he could live another 10 or 12 years.

Still in her 20s, she was inspired. She did not want that same life for herself. She wanted good health in her later years. She quickly stopped smoking and curtailed her weekend drinking with friends. Amanda soon dropped 50 pounds and became a runner.

Another wake-up call

After a layoff, Amanda became a federal contractor, working as a health insurance administrator. "I went to a lot of important places and spoke to a lot of important people about something that's very mundane." She knew that while her career paid the bills and she could continue to make money at it, she was not passionate about health insurance.

She was successful, but as she approached 40, she was rethinking her career path. "My work environment was toxic. I just wasn't happy."

Undoubtedly, there is a helping side to the health insurance industry. Amanda was helping people through her work, but was also wondering, "What am I going to do with the rest of my life?"

And then, her father died, 11 years after his doctor's life-changing advice. "He passed away," Amanda says, "and one day I woke up and said, 'I could die tomorrow, and I'd die unhappy." She couldn't bear the thought. She had made the changes to her physical health to live longer but did not want her life to be unfulfilled. It was time to leave the insurance world.

Helping people help themselves

Amanda found a job as a retail sales associate, moved in with her fiancé to share expenses, and started to determine her next move. Through several months of research and introspection, "all roads pointed to social work," she says. "I like to help people to help themselves, especially when it comes to practical matters; so I thought medical social work would be great." She could quickly envision a level of fulfillment in social work that she had not experienced in her professional life.

She became a private caregiver, in part so she could work with older individuals. "I like that population and I find that it's almost not even work. I'm taking people to appointments, helping them with their house care needs, helping them to do the things they want, and making general conversation. It feels right and I feel a sense of satisfaction in this work." She enrolled in a bachelor's degree program in social work.

Education, the new way

Now, in her 40s, she is older than some of her professors, which has been an adjustment. She has had to re-learn campus culture. "It's interesting, what you don't realize that you don't know. For example: when I went to class the first day, people

"I've learned that I'm very resilient. I'm stronger than I think that I am."

said, 'Tell me what your preferred pronoun is.' And I didn't know what that meant." Luckily, the other students were glad to educate her.

One challenge of being a returning student was coming up to speed on the tools. "I'm tail-end Gen X," she says, "so, although I know how to use technology, there were things that I still needed to learn."

She has learned her way around the Blackboard educational content management system and Discord messaging and social platform, and made the transition from using the Internet instead of a physical library for her research. "It's funny to think back on the card catalog in the libraries of the past," she chuckles.

Her university required her to be on campus in person for her undergrad classes, although hybrid classes were offered during the COVID-19 pandemic. Now, as she begins her graduate studies, her entire curriculum is online.

Amanda says that she thinks older students sometimes make going back more complicated than it needs to be, but she admits to an advantage because she chose not to have children. Some of her younger classmates work full-time jobs and juggle family and children. "All of it is very time-consuming. I couldn't imagine. There are only so many hours in a day."

Yet, she has still demonstrated the capacity to manage multiple priorities. in the middle of her undergraduate program and working as a private caregiver, Amanda was planning her wedding and preparing for her new career.

"I've learned that I'm very resilient. I'm stronger than I think that I am. I have more support than I think that I do, especially from my fiancé (now husband). And that strangers sometimes care more about you than you think that they do. Strangers in school or strangers you care for through your work. So, I've learned a lot."

A lifetime runner

The changes Amanda made in her 20s to improve her health stuck. She continues to run and has become a triathlete and ultramarathoner. "It's hard, but it's not as hard as some people think. Ultramarathoners are usually mostly trail runners, while marathoners are mostly road runners. Trail is a little bit different. It's a lot slower pace.

"Sometimes, because you're going longer distances, you have a lot of time to think about things when you are out in the dark, running by yourself and hoping that you see a flag and you're still going in the right direction.

It takes a big time commitment. It takes knowing what your body can and cannot take. It's a lot of dedication and patience and grace with yourself." These events round out her life and have proven to be beneficial for both her physical and emotional health.

Making a difference

Amanda is now in graduate school part-time at the University of Kentucky, taking classes online. "It's a great program because I can do the work on my own timeline and schedule," she says.

Her dream of a career in social work came true in March 2024 when she became a Social Work Discharge Planner in a skilled nursing facility in Virginia. "I help individuals make a smooth transition from the medical facility to home—in other words, I help them obtain the services they need such as home health care and durable medical equipment (i.e. wheelchairs, walkers, etc.). I also help these individuals file insurance appeals if their coverage ends for their hospitalization, find resources in their area, and other duties. So my career in insurance actually came in handy. This new job is exactly what I was looking for when I originally went back to school. So far, it's hectic, but great and I feel like I can really make a difference here."

Lori Reichel

Taking the Ride

Lori's inner voice urged her on through positions where she felt she didn't quite fit. As an older outsider in her Ph.D. program, she forged ahead and began to establish a challenging academic career. She kept pushing on, now working with college students to give them the skills to be successful health educators while still trying out new opportunities for herself. Lori lives in Upstate New York.

Born and raised on Long Island, Lori Reichel has spent her adult life on the move. Now, she is an assistant professor specializing in health education methodology.

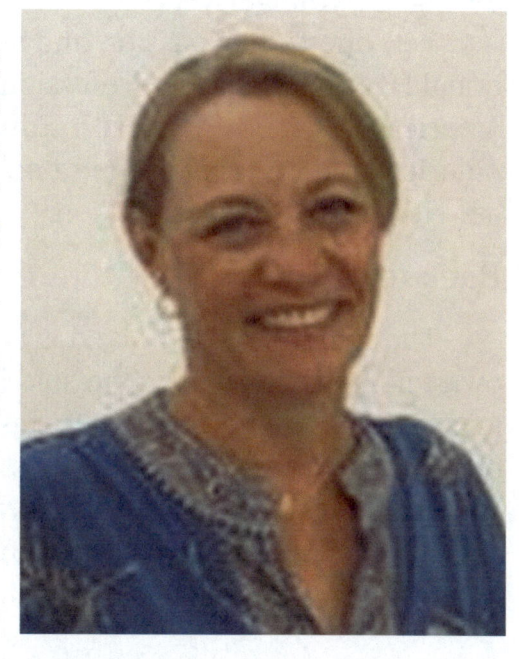

Lori's beginning path was aimed at becoming a teacher, and she took a job as a health education teacher on Long Island which led her to educational administration. But, once she landed the job in administration, she realized that it wasn't her passion and returned to the classroom. Over her 20-year K-12 career, she changed schools or districts several times.

Her 'unorthodox' career path made some people nervous, and some family members and friends didn't understand. In their minds, people chose one career, one employer, and stuck with it until retirement. Making continual changes meant someone couldn't stay employed, and this message was ingrained in her mind from a young age. "I had to figure it out; I had to continuously listen to my inner voice to say, 'What is it that YOU want to do?' And, luckily, I did have some people—angels, I guess—who asked me, 'Hey, why don't you try something new?' This was inspiring and I knew that I wanted to take the ride I'd bought the ticket for."

Lori wanted a life of adventure and opportunity. So, she made her own path. "I'll flat out say, some people think I can't hold a job. And I can definitely hold a job. I just want to make sure I have a job that brings me joy." Satisfaction and joy were never mentioned in early life discussions at school or home during her younger years.

Yet, due to her passion and skill-set, Lori was named National Health Education Professional of the Year in 2010 by the American Alliance for Health Education (now part of SHAPE America) and then given the same honor the following year by her New York state association.

Back to college

Then, in 2011, she walked away from it all and started her own midlife reinvention. She sold her house and used her savings to complete her Ph.D. at Texas A&M University. "It was like being on a trapeze. I had to let go and just trust that I would be successful. It was scary yet exhilarating at the same time."

As an older student, Lori found that returning to college

required adjustments. "I tried to connect with my peers in the classroom, but a lot of them were younger. Several of them went right from their bachelor's to master's programs and they didn't have the life experience that I had."

Overall, Lori wasn't comfortable in the freewheeling social scene of the young adults on campus. "I didn't make any real friends there," she says, "and that's a long time to be in a place and not have even a little bit of a network." She looked for opportunities to meet people and enjoyed the work she did for her PhD, but acknowledges the isolation she often felt as a nontraditional student.

Navigating alone

After graduation, Lori relocated to take a job as an assistant professor at a mid-western university. She looked forward to making a new start and becoming established in the university community. But when she went to an annual physical, doctors found a lump. Lori was diagnosed with two different forms of thyroid cancer. "So, it was my first semester on the faculty, and there I was: new, and not wanting to ruffle too many feathers. But I had to have surgery and needed time off for recovery, shortly after starting the job.

Colleagues rallied to help her through it, but in the end, she never felt that she was part of what she calls the "controlled atmosphere."

She stayed connected with friends from her New York days, but mostly, "I had to figure out how to entertain myself, how to make sure I could be happy. So, I tried different things like hiking and snowshoeing and finding good restaurants. On my birthday, I took myself to a nice restaurant, and had a martini and a great meal."

"It wasn't easy," she says. "I'm not saying that I was depressed. I wasn't. I actually don't mind anything that I did because I know that I'm supposed to be living my life." And it was this solitary time in her life that brought her back to herself to find true happiness and be open to a romantic relationship.

Nearly two years later, Lori met her partner, the man she calls "the love of my life." Now she says of her time in Wisconsin: "It felt lonely sometimes but I've realized that's why I was supposed to be there, to meet him."

Back to New York

They moved to Michigan in late 2019, but the culture was frustrating again. "We looked at the pros and cons—the job paid a similar salary—but I was unhappy in Michigan because I was not respected professionally," she says. "Maybe it's me. Some people say I might be intimidating—not on purpose, but because I want to do the best I can."

In 2022, she and her partner, now retired, moved back to her home state of New York. They found a house they love, and Lori restarted her career once again.

"I never thought I'd return to New York," Lori says, "but it's really interesting to return, to see it through a different lens because of age, or should I say wisdom?"

Lori is now an assistant professor at the State University of New York College at Cortland, with a side practice as a health consultant. She enjoys the flexibility of academia, loves her students, and says she loves being back in New York. "I think I'm finally in a healthier position overall."

Her teaching typically focuses on health education methodology and coordinated school systems, and she occasionally teaches courses on human sexuality. "As I get older, people ask, 'Can you really relate to college students?'" And her answer is, "Yes!"

Lori talks about the way her students share their expe-

Mary Eisenhauer

"Some people say I might be intimidating—not on purpose, but because I want to do the best I can."

riences in class. "It's nice to have this connection because so many young people talk honestly about who they are including sexually... I love that they feel comfortable to tell me about themselves. They feel so comfortable in class because we can talk about anything they have questions about. What I'm learning is that our generation didn't necessarily teach them some of the realities of life," Lori says. One of her missions is to help her students create the "health class that you never had."

If you look online for Lori these days you'll find her podcast, School Health Educators, which is available on YouTube and most streaming platforms, and her former podcast of three years, The Puberty Prof. Continuing her passion for helping children and youth, Lori continues to work with and provide tools for educators and family members. These tools include the books *Common Questions Children Ask About Puberty* and *Tools for Teaching Comprehensive Human Sexuality Education* (co-author) which present topics in plain language accessible to parents, adolescents, and educators. Her newest book, *Tactile Tools for Social Emotional Learning: Activities to Help Children Self-Regulate, PreK-5*, will be released in 2025. Lori also created an online resource where K-12 educators can go to for updated information in their field.

Lori's winding path through jobs and geography led to her

reinvention, and she's satisfied with that. "I'm very blessed. Going through so many moves and different positions—if that got me here, I can't complain and I don't. I took the ride I bought the ticket for!"

Sherry Rigel

The Reinvention Continues

As a young adult, Sherry thought college was out of reach. But now, in midlife, she's a social worker helping older adults, working with therapy dogs, and planning her next amazing transformation. Sherry lives in New Castle, Pennsylvania.

As a child, Sherry Rigel never could have predicted all that she has accomplished.

Her parents divorced when she was in elementary school, and her mother struggled with schizophrenia. "It was a hard life," Sherry says now. "I watched her raise a family despite her mental illness. When my dad left, I watched her figure out,

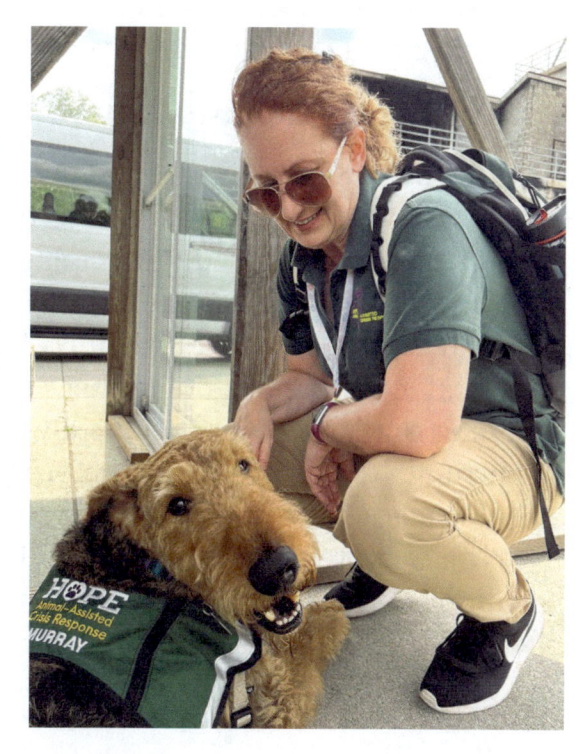

'How am I going to get things done?'" There seemed to be no end to the challenges for her family, financially and otherwise.

When Sherry was a teenager, her mother sent her to live with her older brother's family. "I helped my brother and his wife with their children, but also soon went husband hunting. I wanted to get out of there and didn't know how else to do it. So, I found a wonderful man, moved in with him, got married, and he took care of me. We're still together to this day. He's just a good guy." In him, she found the stability and direction her life had lacked in her younger years, and she was able to see a future for herself.

Sherry and her husband went on to raise a large, blended family, in Pennsylvania. "I'm so grateful for the years I got to be a mom. My husband and I have always budgeted to enable us to live on his salary. It wasn't always easy but we did it. This allowed me to focus on the kids, and when I worked, it paid for the extras like vacations or special things for the kids. They're all financially independent and finding their way in life. Two of them have college degrees. I'm very proud of them."

An unexpected opportunity

In 2008, Sherry homeschooled her youngest daughter, which worked out so well that the education vendor recruited her for a home-based job helping other parents who used the curriculum. She managed message boards on religion, politics, and an online parents' group. "I learned a lot about people and handling situations doing that," she says. The job included traveling to conventions. "It was a wonderful time and a great opportunity to work remotely before 'remote work' was even a thing," she says.

This remote work also enabled her to incorporate an associate's degree program into her schedule, something she had always wanted to pursue. "It was like growing up again when I first went back to college. Even though I was in my 40s, emotionally I felt like I was in my 20s."

Once her youngest daughter graduated from high school, Sherry could see that the education company's management style had changed, and it was time to do something different. Loving the flexibility of working remotely and knowing she needed time for her college classes, she sought positions that would allow her to continue to be home-based. She found that her work for the education company opened doors for her, and her next role was teaching English online to Chinese children. "That was a blast, and again I learned so much about working with children and about the Chinese culture," she says, "but ultimately, I moved on. I'm not a morning person and we worked on China time."

Choosing a new direction

Over the course of four years, she finished her associate's degree. "Cultural anthropology was where my heart was, but let's be honest—there are some doors that close when you get older. I have a husband so I can't run off to Samoa and study a group of people. I needed to take time to figure out a more practical use of my skills."

Sherry says, that as a Gen Xer, she felt she had to find a way to monetize her degree, whatever it turned out to be. "The money wasn't the most important thing for me but I worried that other people would question, 'Why are you spending all of this money on a degree if it's not something that's going to be lucrative?' So, I had to get past that."

She was intrigued by roles in Human Resources and seriously considered HR as a career path. "In HR, you're matching a person and their capabilities to a job that is going to be a good fit for them. There is reward in that. But then I met some people working in HR and realized that you also have to fire people.

There's a lot of paperwork and a lot of legal aspects. So that turned out not to be a field I wanted to pursue."

Crisis response training

Sherry, who had loved dogs all her life, was drawn to a social work program at Slippery Rock University in Pennsylvania that offered a minor in animal-assisted interventions, one of only two such minors in the U.S. She enrolled in the program and quickly learned of the opportunity to join a grant that and become certified by the nonprofit HOPE Animal-Assisted Crisis Response. HOPE, Sherry learned, traveled to disaster scenes, and worked with emergency response teams. What better way to combine her love of supporting people with her love of dogs?

Being certified as a Crisis Response Team leader is "awesome. My role is to liaise between the HOPE canine teams and their handlers and the disaster people or FEMA, and also to care for the canine teams to make sure that the canine handlers can focus on their dogs and on the job that they're there to do." Her work can be as simple as fetching supplies, or as complex as controlling a chaotic scene so that the dogs and handlers can calmly do their work. No two situations are the same, so her role varies from one moment to the next, one response to the next.

Connecting to seniors

Sherry paid for her associate's degree as she went along, refusing to take out student loans until she started her bachelor's program. "Being an older, nontraditional student in a bachelor's program has so many advantages. I had life experiences that the other students didn't have. When we discussed real-life situations in my social work classes, I had so many things to draw from. The younger students weren't in the same situation. I was also in a different place in my life, a more confident

Mary Eisenhauer

> "I've always enjoyed the company of people who are elderly. It's like peeling back an onion... But when you start talking to them, you start finding out the cool things they've done. Their lives can be so interesting."

mindset. But the one thing I didn't have was the same number of years to pay back student loans. So I budgeted to pay tuition as I went along." She blended school time with work in a senior care facility. "I've always enjoyed the company of people who are elderly. It's like peeling back an onion—you see them and they're old. We're all going to be there someday. But when you start talking to them, you start finding out the cool things they've done. Their lives can be so interesting."

So, when it came time for Sherry, then in her 50s, to choose a population to study, she realized that the answer was right in front of her. "I'm old," she laughs, "And I thought that the elderly could appreciate having a social worker that is closer in age to them, rather than having a 25-year-old come in and say, 'Let me help you.' When you're hiring a social worker or a gerontologist, what age do you want to hire? In that case, I think that my age is an asset instead of a detriment."

Crafting her own reinvention

After graduation, Sherry experimented with a job as a protective services investigator for older adults at a large nonprofit agency. "A protective services worker is there to protect the elderly person, first and foremost. It can be complex and multi-faceted, as the worker sees the worst and catches flak from the individual and their family. It's a mentally and emotionally brutal job that requires you to meet in person on a constant basis.

"It became clear that the work/life balance I had expected just wasn't there. Wonderfully, at my age, I know myself well enough and I'm comfortable enough to know when to call it quits."

Sherry still volunteers with HOPE Animal Assisted Crisis Response, helping to screen new canine/handler teams and training them in workshops.

She's also working on her master's degree, pursuing a path that allows her to combine social work with animal-assisted interventions. She'll graduate in May of 2025. "Whatever job happens at that time remains to be seen," Sherry says, "but I know now that Hope Animal-Assisted Crisis Response is where my heart is."

Editor's note: Sherry checked in just before this book went to press, writing: "I've accepted a field placement for next year as a Veterinary Social Worker (intern) at Blue Pearl Pet Hospital. I'm excited to combine my social work major and AAI minor in this new role!"

Business Women

The corporate world often undervalues women in midlife. High achievers can feel that they have been pushed out or passed over for opportunities—but, once they have more time and greater resources, midlife can be the ideal time to live out a dream.

For the women in this section, reinvention meant starting a business after spending the first half of their lives caring for others and/or building careers. The confidence and resilience these women built over decades of personal and professional responsibilities position them well for success on their own terms.

Kavita Ahuja

Prioritize Happiness

Kavita is a Certified (IPEC) Women's Career and Life Transitions Coach and founder of It's My Time Now, a three-month transformational coaching program. She hosts "The Midlife Reinvention," a podcast where she and her guests share "this journey of rediscovery." She lives just outside of Toronto.

Kavita (her name means "poem" in Hindi) Ahuja grew up with an international worldview.

Her grandparents immigrated from India to Kenya to help build railroads in the early 1900s. She was born in Nairobi, but the family moved to Canada when many South Asians were displaced from Kenya in the late 1960s.

Her father, who was an entrepreneur and ran a

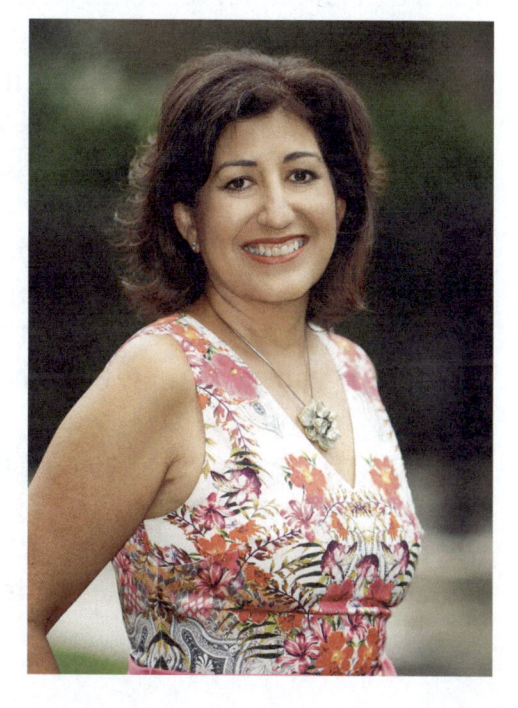

flourishing wheat farm in Kenya, eventually pursued his own real estate business in Canada. Both her parents were her earliest role models.. "I think that's where I got a lot of my entrepreneurial spirit and my adventure in life," she says, citing their strength and determination.

Kavita's parents instilled her and her two sisters with traditional Indian values, encouraging her to get an education as well as to marry and raise a family.

She succeeded in all directions. Kavita and her husband, now married over 30 years, raised two sons. She holds two college degrees, an MBA and a Bachelor of Science in Biology and her successful pharmaceutical sales and marketing career spanned 25 years.

But at about age 50, Kavita felt unfulfilled and restless. A nagging inner voice asked whether the life she'd built was really the one she wanted. "You know: Who are you, really? Are you happy? What do you want to do in the next chapter of your life?"

She thought that by doing this, it would make her happy. But when she did not secure different roles she applied for, she began to question if this is really what was meant for her. She was accustomed to succeeding in all aspects of her life, so at the time, this felt like a big blow to her. And this was the trigger (and later she would learn, the gift) that led her into deep introspection about what would truly make her happy.

Kavita realized that she'd hit a plateau—she wasn't growing anymore—and not just at work. She says her marriage was "great, but the excitement wasn't there anymore." Her sons had grown up, and now they were empty-nesters. She was going through menopause and health changes associated with it. It was time to dig deep and discover what she truly wanted.

"I think I didn't want to regret my life when I look back when I'm 80 years old," she says. "There were things I was passionate about as a child, like writing, and things that I had never

> "The more I push myself without burning out, the more I push myself into things that I never thought I could do, the more I want to keep doing them—and the more that I see that I'm influencing or helping more people."

really explored. And I thought, 'Well, if I'm not going to do it now, when am I going to do this?'"

Facing down fear

Kavita began questioning why some women can reinvent themselves successfully while others remain stuck. She immersed herself in research and learning from such thought leaders as Deepak Chopra, Eckhart Tolle, Oprah Winfrey, Abraham Hicks, and others. She learned about spiritual awakening, the role of fear, energetic alignment and, as Tara Mohr writes, playing bigger.

"Some fears are very valid," Kavita says. "They are there to keep you safe, like the fear of 'Am I going to make enough money to do whatever I need to do?'"

But she also learned that fear of failure, judgment, or even success can hold women back from transition and growth. She conquered her fears through her inner beliefs, visualization, and the knowledge that she had so much more to offer the world with skills and passions that were still untapped.

She realized that, like many women, she had been trying to please others rather than prioritize her own needs. "Ultimately if we want to be happy, then we have to follow our hearts," she says now. And Kavita now realizes that the pivotal moment when she did not get that promotion at work was a gift.

She stresses the need to celebrate accomplishments and know that success motivates more growth. Pushing herself to do things she would never have believed she could do—such as podcasting—also helps her influence and help more people. "The more I push myself without burning out, the more I push myself into things that I never thought I could do, the more I want to keep doing them—and the more that I see that I'm influencing or helping more people."

Friends and family

Kavita acknowledges her strong support system, starting with her husband, whom she calls her biggest champion. Her adult sons encourage her, listening to her podcast and giving feedback. But not everyone understood Kavita's transition. Some friends and family, especially those who have traditional values, questioned her change, saying, "Everything seems perfect, so why would you rock the boat?"

Kavita says this judgment is common when women diverge from the traditional path, and she says that, in her case, they were coming from a place of care and concern, not necessarily criticism. For most of her life, Kavita had felt pressure to meet external expectations but finally prioritized her own fulfillment and happiness when she turned 50.

Ripples of success

With her husband's full support, Kavita made the leap to become a coach and launched "The Midlife Reinvention" podcast that helps other women make midlife transitions.

Kavita says that women should listen to that inner voice telling them that something needs to change. "It's all about the timing. My coaching practice, It's My Time Now, is about having the courage to take the first step. And if you don't know how to do it, then ask for help."

Her own career reinvention catalyzed her transformation, and the ripples have brought her calmness, healthier habits, and greater spirituality. She started meditating, doing yoga, and getting more in touch with her Eastern roots. She focuses on living in the present moment with gratitude. She travels.

This has led to increased energy and zest for life. Her marriage, family relationships, and friendships have all benefited from her internal shift.

The next step

Kavita draws inspiration from her clients' profound transformations, from career shifts to lifestyle changes to pursuing education later in life. Her own next step is to write a book and expand her reach to help more women.

"I think I'm more energized than I have been in a long time," Kavita says. "If you're happy with what you're doing, if you are surrounded by people that support you, and if you're helping people and see the transformations that you can have in people's lives—it's so fulfilling and energizing that it just leads into other aspects of your life."

Marie Ambusk

The Root of the Problem

Marie's roots are in corporate finance, but these days it's the roots of trees that concern her. She's building a tech startup on her passion for understanding how to help trees thrive in the urban landscape where we live Marie lives in central Vermont.

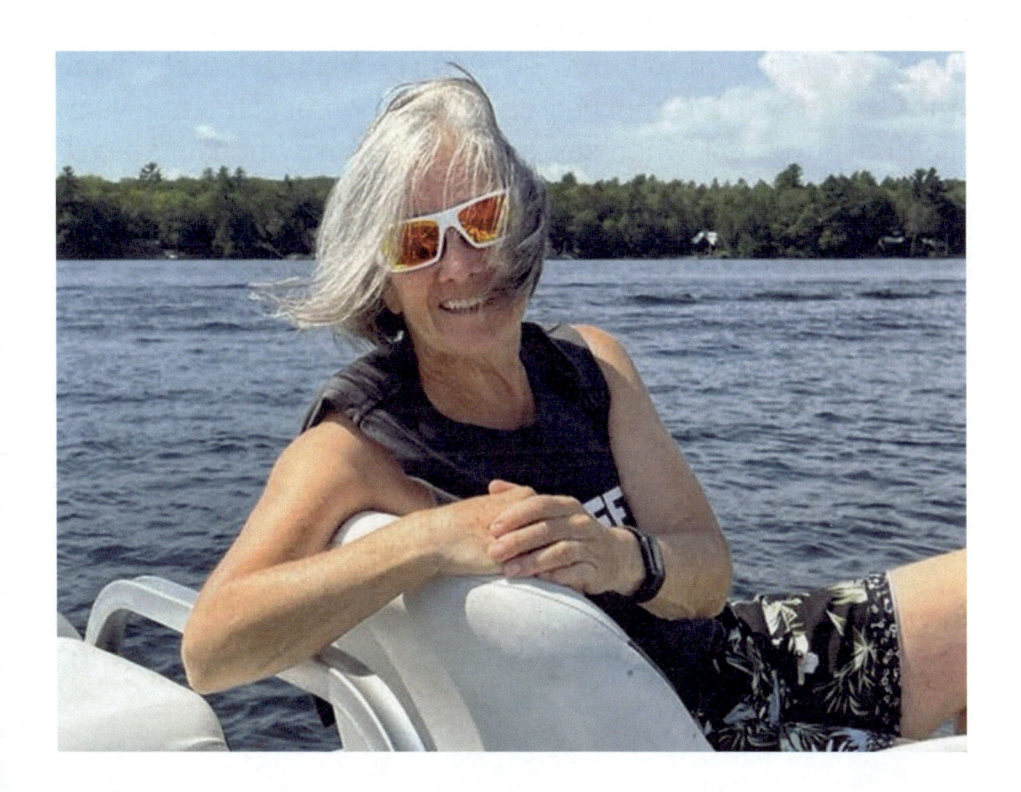

> "I've come to believe that anything, any problem, I don't even care what it is, can be solved using science and technology, with a good idea, a lot of work, and a little luck."

Marie Ambusk built a successful 40-year career managing complex accounting systems, including 28 years at IDX Systems (now GE Healthcare). She had always enjoyed her work and her colleagues, but at the same time, was happy to retire early and move on to a new adventure—whatever that adventure would be. Her unexpected reinvention began a few years before retirement when she moved into a new housing development.

Dead trees grew the idea that became her aha moment. Shortly after moving into the development, Marie saw that the newly planted street trees had died in a terrible windstorm. The city arborist blamed "root collar disorder," a problem that occurs when the roots of a young tree circle around the base of the trunk inside a too-small nursery pot and strangle it. The landscaper said he would just replace the trees with whatever others he got from the supplier: "Lady, you get what you get."

Marie didn't understand what was happening. "I can't accept that the trees are just going to continue to be produced with bad roots and die early when they should live 80 to 100 years or more. I thought, 'Well, someone should fix this problem, and nobody was interested in fixing it.' So, I decided that person would be me."

On a volunteer basis, she would spend as much as 10 hours on one tree, carefully digging around the roots to diagnose the problem. "After doing this work on trees for a couple of days I went to bed, I closed my eyes and all I could see was these roots, terrible roots underground. And when I woke up literally from a dream, I thought, 'I need a crystal ball to see what's in the ground so that I can determine if there's a problem that I can fix, or if it's beyond my help.'"

Her new interest in trees led Marie to become a certified master gardener, as well as train with Vermont's Stewardship of the Urban Landscape (SOUL) Tree Steward Program. SOUL offers courses on tree identification, biology, and planting; resource assessment; landscape design; and conservation planning, all of which proved valuable to her research. "I decided I would lead a volunteer project to help people understand how to take care of these trees. And I'm still leading project TREEage today, 15 years later."

All of this education raised Marie's awareness. There were unhealthy trees not only in her neighborhood but throughout her town. She decided more needed to be done. "It started me on this path to educate myself about how trees live, how they die, or why they die," she says, "and what, if anything, we can possibly do to influence their ability to thrive in our neighborhoods like this, in the urban landscape where people live?"

She learned that the problem may have started at the nurseries where young trees were grown in containers, calling the growers "the root of the problem": "You know what your house plants look like when you pull them out of a container and their roots are all wrapped around? Well, that's what happens to the trees and these containers."

A career in problem-solving

Her career at IDX had given Marie the tools to solve problems with technology and take on complex challenges. "We were a small software company doing amazing things that no one had ever done before. Growing up in that environment... I've come to believe that anything, any problem, I don't even care what it is, can be solved using science and technology, with a good idea, a lot of work, and a little luck."

With this in mind, she first investigated using ground penetrating radar (GPR) in 2010. Initial testing was unsuccessful, but after years of exploring other technologies, she returned to Geophysical Survey Systems Inc (GSSI) to find their technological advancements offered hope to support her vision. "I'm so grateful for the scientists at GSSI who embrace innovation and this novel use of GPR. They are among my mentors who encourage me with cautious optimism and pragmatic goals to keep moving onward."

Marie holds a US Utility Patent for the innovation. Her tech startup, TreesROI™, is developing INSIGHT™, a 3D GPR Tree CT system to assess and grade the quality of container-grown tree roots. INSIGHT™ is a non-destructive tool for growers, developers, municipalities, and tree asset owners to give quality grading and tree care recommendations for correcting serious root problems before planting (if correctable).

TreesROI™ is a 2024 awardee of a coveted Small Business Innovation Research (SBIR) grant funded by the National Science Foundation (NSF). With seed funding and substantial progress, they enthusiastically face the hurdles ahead.

Personal challenge

Marie's finance career combined valuable skills in analytics, systems thinking, and tenacity, along with her extensive tree biology training, to complete her mission. It turned out that her approach allowed her to connect usually siloed jobs and information to make the concept work.

"It's funny, they call me the outsider," she says. "Really, I'm not a certified arborist. I'm not a scientist. I'm not a programmer. There are so many things that I'm not—and yet they'll say, 'Well, isn't it interesting that an outsider would be the one to come to our industry and solve the problem?' So, it's just a funny reality, I guess."

Marie has a long history of trusting science and technology to solve problems. In addition to her career at IDX, and in addition to her work with the trees, she found herself having to trust a team of medical professionals to treat the brain tumor she was diagnosed with in 2014. It was the fight of her life as she underwent surgery and extensive rehab therapy, unable to predict survival and quality of life after treatment.

Marie reflects, "I remember thinking I wanted to return to our research project. And that if I could get through treatment and recovery, I wanted to use technology—the kind of technology they used to scan my brain and map the tumor that helped to save my life—to scan and map tree roots so we can understand what's going on and help to save their lives."

While she still struggles with some lasting effects of the acquired brain injury from ten years ago, Marie feels she has found her life's purpose: grow better trees. "I'm grateful that most people are surprised to learn about this part of my story. And, hopefully, I will live long enough to achieve this big goal."

Never settle

For women considering major life changes, Marie quotes Ellen Johnson Sirleaf, Liberian president and the first female elected as a head of state in Africa: "If your dreams do not scare you, they are not big enough." She also echoes a quote sometimes attributed to Theodore Roosevelt: "People don't care how much you know until they know how much you care."

By applying her skills and knowledge to her passion project, Marie has created a legacy that will literally, and figuratively, change the landscape of communities for generations to come.

Kimchi Chow

Stand Up, Show Up

Kimchi immigrated to the United States to find a better life, but it took a financial crisis to move her to seek inner peace. Her passion for helping other Asian immigrants led her to coaching. Kimchi lives in San Jose, California.

Kimchi Chow, the founder and CEO of Asian Women of Power, is a certified Positive Intelligence Coach, specializing in cultural integration coaching and empowering Asian American women. It is a journey she has walked herself.

Kimchi was 20 when she immigrated to the United States. She brought with her the cultural expectations of her native Vietnam.

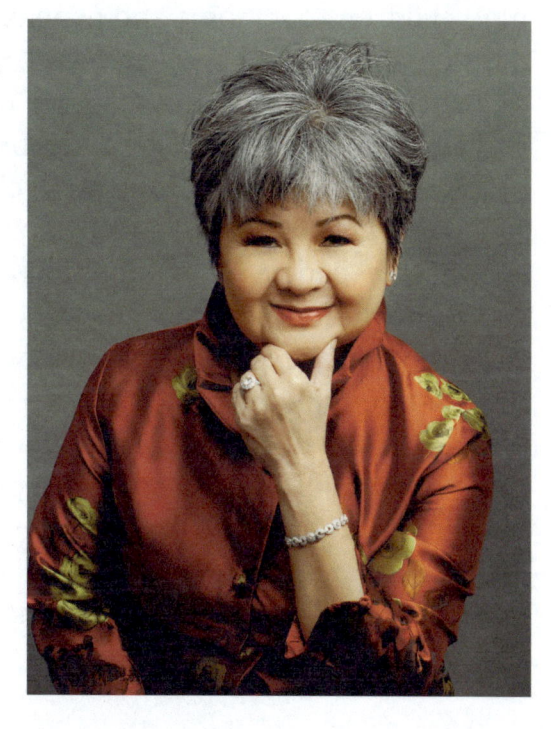

Her mother, a businesswoman with nine children, is her role model. "She had only a fifth-grade education," Kimchi says, "but she knew how to manage and work with people." During the 60s and 70s, most small businesses in Vietnam gave credits to their regular clients so they could encourage more sales. Her mother, with great people skills, knew how to create trust so all of her vendors would sell her fabric and merchandise on credit. And that's how her mother was able to create the largest fabric store in the city where they lived with a minimum start-up cost.

Earn your own money

After the family immigrated, the older kids went to night school to learn English. When her mother interviewed for an assembly line job, her brother went along to translate. "Her English skill was just enough to say, 'yes' or 'no'," Kimchi says now, but the supervisor recognized her mother's immigrant "working mentality" and hired her on the spot. Immigrants were known for their strong work ethic and being resourceful. With nine children to support and expenses to cover, her immigrant mother was an ideal employee.

Later in life, Kimchi asked her mother why she hadn't just stayed home, keeping house and looking after the younger children who were still in elementary school. Her mother's answer: "It's important for women to be able to earn their own money so that they can be independent of a man."

Kimchi later applied that same mindset to her own marriage. "I wanted to call the shots. I was married, I had two children, a good job, a big house, two cars—all those things, and, actually, I was not happy in my marriage." She thought having her own income would garner respect from her husband and his family. But her husband, who immigrated from Taiwan when he was 10 years old, was raised in a traditional family and his mother never worked outside the home. "It's a different expec-

"Once you are clear about what's important for you? The experienced coach will guide you to the action."

tation," she acknowledges.

She describes her husband as "very conservative, a low risk taker. I'm a high risk taker and I make decisions very quickly. This difference is a real challenge so I was not happy," she says, "and I thought, 'Okay, there must be something wrong with me. I need to find a way to be happy." She began what she calls a journey of discovering myself. Her conclusion: compromise, and picking battles carefully.

"Nobody can give you happiness, only you. You can bring yourself happiness and happiness is internal, not external. I said, 'Okay. So, my husband cannot make me happy. My parents cannot make me happy. I need to do it myself, my way. I need to find things that I'm happy to do and that I love to do. And, once I recognize that nothing can stop me."

Not a stay-at-home mom

It took time for Kimchi to fully embrace this concept and understand how to make herself happy. Her early career was focused on quality engineering for tech firms. When her children were in high school, she decided to take a break after the company where she worked was acquired. At the time, she thought 'I'm done with working! Let me stay home and be a mom while I figure out what happens next."

She had tried staying home for a year when her first child was born. "I was miserable all day. I'd just talk baby talk and hang out with all the other women who were at home. And I realized that I needed to be able to communicate intelligently." She managed only six months at home with her second child. "I definitely know for sure I'm not a typical housewife. So that's it. I gave up on the idea."

Kimchi acknowledges that "My ideal situation is challenging my brain and also being able to make money... My mom's voice is always in my head, saying that if you want to be in control, make your own money."

So, she decided to start her own business, parlaying a few rental properties she and her husband owned into her own property management company. She used her retirement accounts to build a portfolio in real estate, securities, and business investments. While this was a tremendous experience, Kimchi learned some painful lessons in the 2008 recession. These lessons took a toll on her marriage and her outlook, leaving her rudderless and discouraged. "She realized she had spent years keeping busy—very busy." The reason is because I was not happy inside," she says.

Empowering Asian-American women

Kimchi says her "light-bulb moment" was in 2014 when she became an unpaid coach for several entry-level Landmark Education leadership programs, an opportunity that came to her from her professional network. "I talked to clients only two times and they were able to turn around their relationships," she says. "I was so happy—I said, 'This is exciting. I can do this forever.'" Soon after, she trained to become a certified life coach and turned her new passion into a business. Through the process of becoming certified, she realized that she needed to forgive herself for the chaos caused by her financial losses and the toll it all took on her marriage.

As an extension of her coaching business and with her immigrant experience at the forefront of her mind, Kimchi started a podcast, "Asian Women of Power," in May 2018. She interviewed powerful Asian-American women and men and shared her own experiences as an immigrant dealing with the conflicting cultural values of East and West. The podcast focused on helping her audience, whether recent immigrants or those from families who have been in the United States for generations, "to speak up, to stand up, and to show up powerfully and confidently."

Kimchi's advice for Asian women who are considering making big changes in their lives is to begin by finding a life coach who has a deep cultural understanding for their fears, concerns and family expectations, and who has several decades of life experience. With that mutual understanding, an experienced coach can help expand their perspectives about life and about what really matters. "When they find the right coach, clients can achieve long lasting joy, happiness and fulfillment."

Marie Gettel-Gilmartin

Ask for What You Deserve

Marie started life with multiple surgeries and became a target for school bullies. Now, she uses the resilience she learned to power her business and mentor other women. Marie lives in Portland, Oregon.

Marie Gettel-Gilmartin says "I have realized, especially in my later years, that my whole life has been one of resilience." It's her favorite word.

Marie was born in Portland, Oregon, and she learned resilience early on. "I was actually born with a cleft lip and palate, and so my whole childhood was full of multiple surgeries and

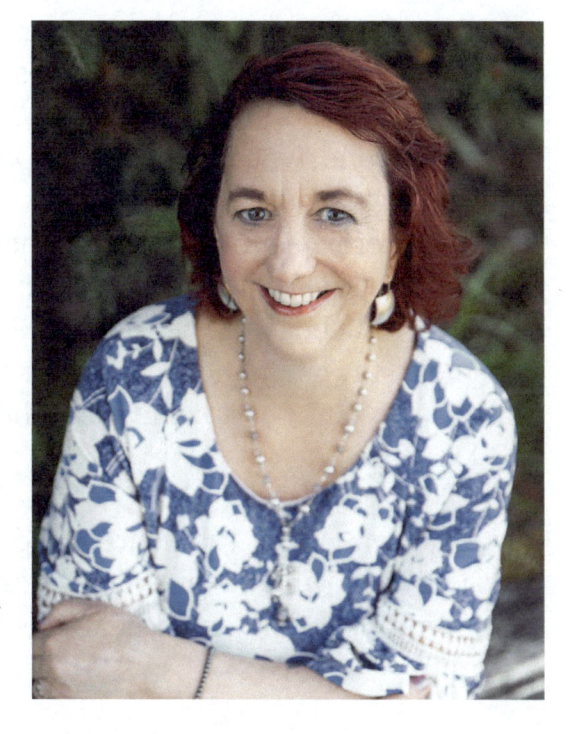

> "I like the fact that I've been able to build a business grounded firmly in my values. It is very freeing—but on the other hand, it's also hard."

some bullying in middle school." Having the stress of ongoing medical issues and feeling different from her peers taught her early in life how to navigate challenges.

But once Marie graduated from Pacific Eastern University in Tacoma, Washington, she was ready to take wing. She spent three years in the 1980s teaching English in Japan. She met her future husband, who is British, in Japan, and together they traveled throughout Asia.

They returned to Oregon and married. "He wanted to write his novel," Marie remembers, "so I told him I would support him for a year." He became the "household manager" and eventually became a stay-at-home dad to their three sons. "I realized that I liked to go out to work and I had the marketable skills."

Corporate career

That was more than three decades ago, and they're still married. Meanwhile, Marie built a career at an environmental consulting firm that lasted nearly as long. "I started out as the temporary receptionist, and then I found out they had an editing department, so I was hired as a junior editor there."

The company "re-engineered" its structure several times during her time there, combining regions and restructuring its staff. A female mentor guided Marie, and "within a couple of years, I was promoted to be the supervisor of the department, leading all these women who were older than me."

She rose through the company to become manager of the northwest publications department for 13 years and reinventing herself into a communications manager for sustainability and corporate citizenship, but then the entire company was acquired by another corporation. She was offered a choice: severance or stay on in another role.

But staying meant that she would no longer be working in communications. She didn't want to work for a company that would keep the corporate communications officer, who led a "really toxic and dysfunctional" department.

Again, she faced a toxic work environment that pitted her against a male boss who had less management experience than she had, something that women in midlife often face. "I'm very respectful, but I speak my mind. So, I got laid off."

She was asked to continue for a month to finish a website, which was a difficult experience: "I had to promote the company that had just laid me off and deal with my horrific boss who had 'analysis paralysis' and couldn't make decisions." Three months later, the company asked her to become a contractor.

She applied for more than 100 jobs. "I had a number of interviews," she says, but believes that age discrimination kept her from finding a new opportunity.

Finding fertile ground

"So that is how my business was born. "I decided to open up shop, and I came up with the name Fertile Ground Communications because I wanted to find my fertile ground."

On the advice of a friend, Marie saw a therapist for a few months just before the COVID-19 pandemic. "She helped me to get from 'I have to start a business' to 'I get to start a business.' I came to the realization that there was a reason why I didn't get any of those other jobs that I applied for because I was meant to do this."

She and her husband had some savings to fall back on, and he took a job in healthcare to help support the household. "I felt like I had a gift. A lot of people go into the hole when they start their businesses, and I haven't had to do that."

Marie wears many hats at Fertile Ground: founder and principal, but also writer and strategic communications coach, leadership communications coach, marketing and communications auditor, content creator, and strategist.

Among her clients is the Cultural Advocacy Coalition of Oregon; as their contracted communications manager, she produces public-facing content about the state's arts, culture, history, heritages, and humanities. She specializes in "translating technical language into engaging, accessible content."

Marie misses the collaboration she enjoyed in previous jobs, and she is looking forward to building her team. During the pandemic, she highlighted historically excluded voices on her two podcasts.

Never settle

In a March 2023 article for LinkedIn Pulse on International Women's Day, Marie wrote about 'Women Who Have Inspired Me to Ask for What I Deserve." She mentions her mother and sister, her fifth-grade teacher, and her college feminist theology professor. But she also names several businesswomen who mentored and encouraged her. In her introduction to the article, she writes:

Mary Eisenhauer

"I'm grateful to the women in my life who have taught me to stand up for myself and ask for what I deserve. I have worked with, interviewed, and known so many incredible women in my life... but I pay homage to these women on International Women's Day who taught me not to settle."

Tracy Vontélle Green and Nancey Flowers Harris

Build What You Need

Tracy Vontélle Green was born into a bustling Harlem family. Nancey Flowers Harris is the first in her large Jamaican family to be born in the U.S. Together, Tracy and Nancey drew on the lessons they learned from their strong mothers and created a groundbreaking company to offer fashionable eyewear especially for people of color. Their company, Vontélle, is based in New York.

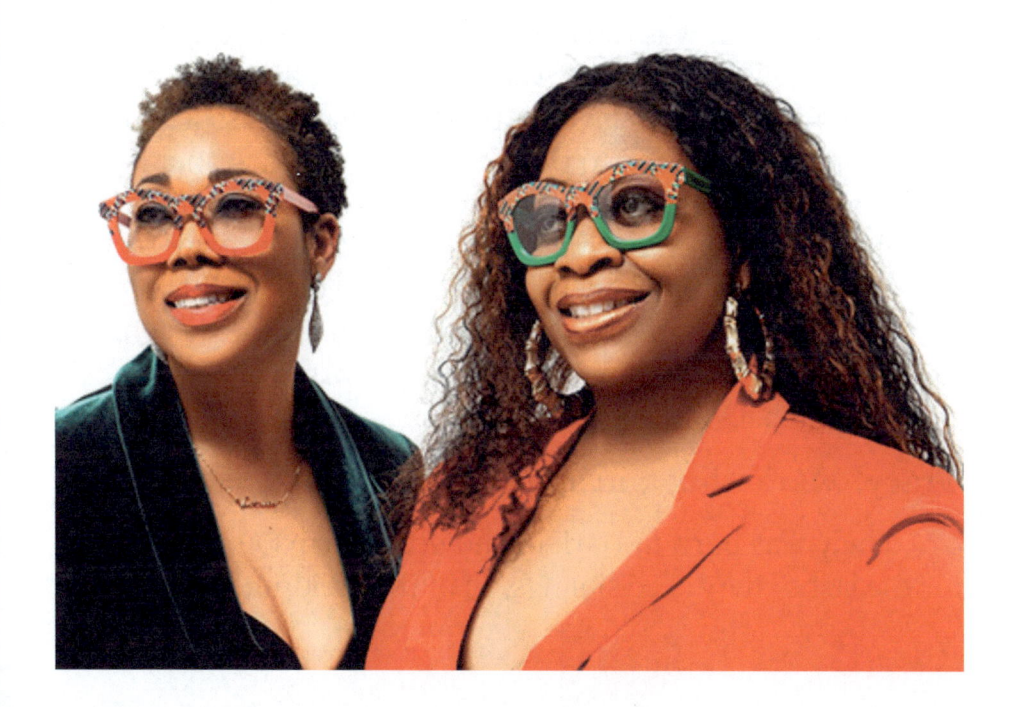

Losing expensive sunglasses can be an annoyance, but for Tracy Vontélle Green and Nancey Flowers Harris, it was the catalyst for their reinvention.

Friends since college, Tracy and Nancey had spent decades in corporate jobs and were both ready for something new. In early 2019, Nancey paid almost $1,000 for custom sunglasses and promptly lost them. By summer, Tracy had bought and lost a pair of her own. They were frustrated not only at the cost but because the products didn't fit them properly.

"You have to realize people of different ethnicities look different," Tracy says "We have different constructs. We have different features in our faces, the shapes of our heads. The glasses we saw on the market were largely designed for Caucasian features. And now I think people are starting to notice because we're saying it."

They founded their company Vontélle (in French, it means "there she goes") that year. "I saw the business opportunity," Nancey says. "We had two things in mind when we wanted to do this business. One of them was to purchase glasses from someone of color. That was the big thing. And then, the other was to find glasses with patterns." Their website defines the realization of those goals: "Each of our products and accessories is designed and handcrafted to pay homage to our African ancestry with traditional colors and patterns that channel our African, Caribbean, and Latin heritage. Our patterns use many textiles and designs from highly identifiable, recognizable, and respected materials like mud cloth and kente cloth. These designs are tailored to empower humanity to see the world through a cultural and global lens."

Tracy: Marketing and style

Tracy was born in Harlem and grew up in Queens. Except for the last of her three siblings, all of the children were born at

Mary Eisenhauer

"I wanted to get into business because I knew that business was the way to change my life."

~ Tracy Vontélle Green

home, with her grandmother as nurse midwife. "My mom and my grandmother were like our rocks," Tracy says. Her stepfather was in the military. She describes her family tree as "very diverse and mixed." Her mother is still studying their genealogy, and the family is learning that their lineage includes African, Scottish, and Spanish threads.

Tracy is the first college graduate in her family. She acknowledges the influence of the strong women in her family. Her grandmother raised the children while her mother worked. Her aunt, a U.S. Marine, urged her to go to college.

Her mother worked in marketing, and one of Tracy's first jobs was interning at the company where her mother was a secretary. Tracy was enrolled in a business high school in Manhattan, so she'd take the train in from Queens to attend school and then finish her day at her internship job. "That was my first time seeing what work life was like," she says. "I wanted to get into business because I knew that business was the way to change my life."

It was also where she realized that fashion could be important to her success. "You're in Manhattan, you see all these women in suits with big shoulder pads and pumps... No one that I that I interacted with on a daily basis dressed like that, right?

I would see my mom dressed up for work and she was fabulous. Her blue eye shadow! She was fashionable. When you went into her office, all the women looked very professional, and they had briefcases and they had suits. I was like, I'm going to have a briefcase and a suit. To this day, I have to say—and Nancey teases me—I love wearing suits."

Nancey: Deep roots in success

Nancey's mother immigrated from Jamaica to Brooklyn in 1970 and Nancey was born the next year, the youngest and first American-born child in her large family.

"My mom is my role model," Nancey says. "She took a chance, coming to this country. She left her entire family to begin a new life in this country, and she sacrificed herself in doing so." When Nancey's father died ten years later, her mother brought the rest of her family, including Nancey's grandparents and two uncles, to America. "I knew that no matter what came, I had to be successful because she really worked very hard."

Nancey's mother, with only a high school education, worked as a nanny and hotel maid. She made sure that Nancey's older sisters went to college. "They set the road map for me; I knew that the way for me to be successful was to go to college and do well. I have other family members who are doctors and nurses. They've all laid the foundation for me to be where I am today."

Ready for a new adventure

Nancey and Tracy met at Morgan State University, where Tracy was working on a BA in political science and Nancey was doing a BA in mass communications/journalism.

After undergrad, Tracy completed her MPA from John Jay College (CUNY) in fiscal policy and finance management. Her first job out of graduate school was as a budget analyst in the

> "Celebrate each win, no matter how small. There are moments when things won't go well, but you have to have faith. If you have a road map and a blueprint, then things will unfold. Things don't happen overnight. It takes five years to become an overnight sensation."
>
> ~ Nancey Flowers Harris

mayor's Office of Management and Budget during the Giuliani administration. She worked for the city's Department of Education and Department of Human Resources and Management and later became chief financial officer of a healthcare company.

Nancey's first job was as an administrative assistant at Architectural Digest. She soon discovered her passion for sales and embarked on a successful career in the field. She started as a sales manager at Viacom and advanced to sales management roles at Black Enterprise magazine, BET Networks, and Wendy Williams Productions.

To jumpstart their business, Nancey bought tickets to the largest eyewear expo in the world, which was being held in Paris. Tracy reluctantly took time off from the hospital, and they spent four days immersed in the industry, walking about 20,000 steps a day as they joined 37,000 attendees in the massive exhibit halls. They saw few other people of color. They came away exhausted, but knowledgeable and with a manufacturer for their products. "Once we went to that Paris show and we saw the expo and learned so much, we realized that we really had to come out strong," Tracy says.

The little project

In December 2019, Tracy became ill with a rare form of diabetes while on an overseas trip with her husband and son. She took a month off from her job. "I was just getting my health back," Tracy says. "Nancey and I were still kind of talking about the eyewear business, doing measurements and research. And then COVID hit in March."

During the pandemic lockdown, Nancey was able to work from home. Tracy, still ill, struggled every day to go into her office in Brooklyn, where infection rates continued to soar. "I was still at work, trying to pay traveling nurses and help keep the hospital running, when half of my team became sick with COVID. I was the only one at the hospital, making payroll." Her health continued to decline, and she lost 40 pounds.

Her manager finally offered to let her work from home some days. Instead, Tracy's family urged her to quit. "My husband said, 'Take a year off work on your little project'—he kept calling it a 'little project'—and I said 'Okay'." And this year not only allowed her to focus on that 'little project', but it also enabled Tracy to manage her health.

It was the beginning of their company. "So now I'm 100% full on, driving Nancey nuts, but it worked out because I think that year that I was home, we got the business up and running... I was able to take all those years of experience and throw it into the business. My husband doesn't call it a little project anymore."

Growing their dream

Each woman brought her own strengths to the project. "We know our wheelhouses," Nancey says. Tracy learned the financial side of the business, working with banks and sales channels. Meanwhile, Nancey studied the process of how to make glasses and learned technical drawing to do their first designs. "It wasn't that difficult for me because I also have an artistic background like I always love, love, love to draw and do presentations so that it was it was like second nature to me."

Nancey's experience in publishing and manufacturing is evident in every aspect of Vontélle, from the intricate "pattern inside pattern" packaging to the glasses' design. "I wanted our presentation to speak for itself. When people unbox our glasses, I want them to feel the full experience and see the detail and passion we pour into each design. That passion extends to all our endeavors. My previous roles in publicity, marketing, sales, and publishing have all led to this moment and shaped where we are today."

Nancey says they are also growing their team. "It's hard to find people who are invested in what you're doing and believe in what you're doing. We don't want lip service. We want you to actually do the work and prove to us that you are in this for the long haul with us so that we can all grow together."

Tracy says their next goal is to get more distribution. They've had some successes, she says, including an insurance plan that wants to allow its clients to use their plans to pay for glasses. "There have been obstacles," Tracy says, "but I think we just keep saying, 'Okay, let's do this little piece. How do we fix it? We're not trying to do everything at the same time, and we have people who help us do things right. Once something comes up, we talk about it." Usually, one or the other of them can make a call. "Literally, by the next day, it's usually fixed."

Do the first step

Nancey's advice to would-be entrepreneurs? "Celebrate each win, no matter how small. There are moments when things won't go well, but you have to have faith. If you have a road map and a blueprint, then things will unfold. Things don't happen overnight. It takes five years to become an overnight sensation."

Tracy agrees. "Just do the first step... I don't think you have to have the answers. We didn't have the answers. When we went to Paris, we had no answer. So, I would tell that person, young or old or whatever, don't be fearful. Just take that little step; chip away at it. Do the first thing, and then you'll do the second thing., and then, before you know it, you're four years in and you have an eyewear company."

"As black women, we don't know fear," Nancey says. That's not part of our vocabulary. We take chances every day just being who we are. You have to be resilient. You have to be strong, like Tracy said. She asks for everything and she's not afraid to stand up for what she believes in and what she wants. And that is so important."

Tracy often cites Nelson Mandela: "It always seems impossible until it's done."

Editor's note: Vontelle checked in just before this book went to press, writing: "Vontélle is the first Black Women Owned Eyewear company to design a collection for America's Best 900+ stores nationwide and obtain a licensing agreement with Nickelodeon Paramount to create a children's line (also sold online at Amazon & Walmart).

"In addition, Saks Fifth Avenue carries a curated collection online, and we designed a commemorative 50th Hip Hop Collection. Notably, we have partnered with VSP insurance plan, Shop Bop and Sam's Club to sell our top sellers...

"Vontélle Eyewear collaborated with National Vision, Inc., the nation's second largest optical retailer on a new frame collection. The limited-edition Official by Vontélle frames is sold in all 900+ America's Best Contacts & Eyeglasses retail locations, marking the first nationwide retail availability for Vontélle frames. Official by Vontélle launched in February 2024...

"Most importantly, Vontélle has partnered with WIN (Women In Need) a New York City organization with over 14 homeless shelters and we provide free eye exams and donate prescription eyewear to men, women, and families in need...

"Vontélle has been in several magazines: InStyle, LA Fashion Magazine, Forbes, Essence, Black Enterprise, Vision Monday, etc. In addition, we also have celebrities such as Queen Latifah in her hit show The Equalizer in the Moroccan Wayfarer Burgundy; Janelle James on Abbott Elementary in Sahara Addax & Pharaoh Giraffe Sunglasses; Chef Marcus Samuelsson of Red Rooster Restaurants & TV personality in Keys to Kenya Blue; Pauletta Washington, Actress in Hulu series Reasonable Doubt, Tiffany Whitlow, Reality Star of Love & Marriage Huntsville on OWN, Steve Harvey, the Comedian, Actor and Radio & TV personality in Acacia Aviators, Tamika Scott from R&B group Xscape and so many more."

Healing and Helping

Decades of adulthood bring women a wealth of experiences—and sometimes heartache. Serious illness, loss of beloved family members, or unexpected life changes cause significant shifts in the lives of many midlife women.

In midlife, we can have the wisdom and resilience to navigate heartache, reinvent ourselves after loss, and even go on to help others address their own challenges.

The women in this section look at needs around their communities and strive to meet those needs in a variety of ways. As they've reinvented themselves in service to others, they enable others to reinvent themselves.

Jackie Capers Brown

Find Your Spiritual Center

Jackie built a thriving career in the hospitality industry despite the life-changing adversities of losing both parents by 19 and the unexpected loss of her only son. Now, she shares the insights, habits, skills, and strategies she's learned to help others connect to the wisdom and power within their soul to embrace their authentic self, enhance their well-being, and achieve uncommon success. She lives in Columbia, South Carolina.

Jackie Capers Brown brings the skills she used to build a successful corporate career to help other women discover and embrace their authentic wholenesss.

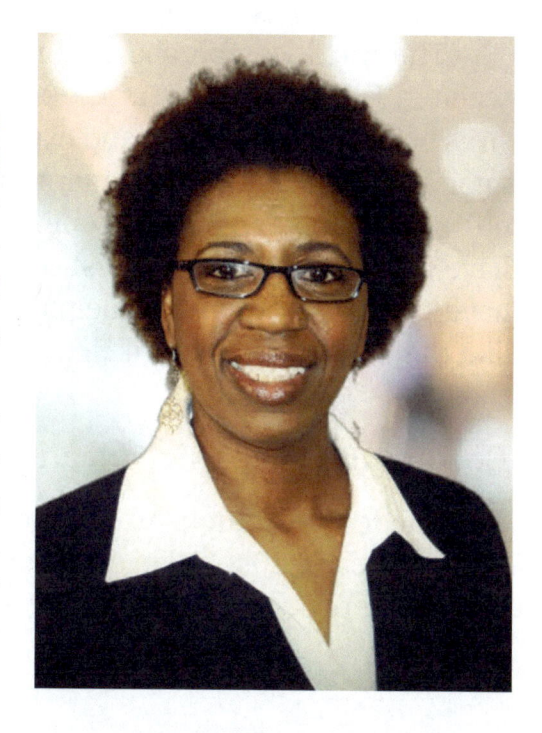

Jackie says her values came from her parents, who, who—although neither was a high-school graduate—raised their large family in a working-class household in Columbia, South Carolina. "At a young age, I was being trained to think above and beyond my circumstances and to not allow the circumstances to define me," she says.

As the eighth of ten siblings, she also picked up some people skills: "One of the most important things about growing up in a large family is that it trained me to interact with different people."

Her mother was her first role model. "The reason why I admired my mom so was because she was always giving to other people in our neighborhood, even though she had limited means."

Jackie's Girl Scouts leader gave her an early glimpse of leadership. "She allowed me to help her run some of our meetings. And that's when I began to get the taste of leadership at the age of eight and nine. My Girl Scout experience helped me develop the confidence to audition for roles in my elementary school plays, and when I was chosen for a role, my ability to speak on stage with confidence reflected the leadership skills I was developing as a Girl Scout."

The third woman she admired most was her third-grade teacher. Jackie says that, at the time, the civil rights movement "was beginning to expand and explode." Her teacher "would remind our class that "Your generation is going to have more opportunities than any other generation preceding you, and you have to not only do your best in your education but also you have to pay it forward by helping the people behind you just like the leaders in the civil rights movement are doing for you today."

Becoming a recognized leader

The lessons stuck. After experiencing a spiritual awakening in her early 20s, Jackie embraced radical forgiveness, which helped her to begin the process of transforming her relationship with herself, her past and present and with those who were the source of the experiences that had led to her harboring anger, bitterness and resentments in her heart.

Her spiritual awakening led to her ending an abusive relationship and moving with her two children to temporarily live with her older sister Glendia. She was hired by the Columbia Marriott hotel as a full-time housekeeper. A month after her probationary period ended, she was promoted to the housekeeping administrative position. The increase in pay enabled her to secure another apartment for her and her two children.

Once she was confident in her new role, she says, "I went into my manager's office one day and asked him to teach me some of his duties... so that I could begin to prepare myself to become a housekeeping manager with the company. My manager was young and ambitious. He wasn't threatened by my bold ask."

Three years later, she transferred to Marriott's Courtyard division as a housekeeping supervisor. Seven months after that, she was promoted and became the housekeeping manager. And five years later, she had managed every department in the hotel, secured five promotions and was about to take on her first of five GM roles she would attain during her corporate career.

Jackie rejects other people's assumptions of what she might achieve based on her race or economic status. "I could not allow the circumstances or even people's limiting perspectives of me as a single mom living on government assistance and food stamps to define me... I decided that I would no longer agree with anyone's opinion of me unless it aligned with my soul's truth."

Jackie says that, as she got older, she "became more self-aware and more understanding of consciousness and awareness. That's when I realized that they were projecting their own limitations on me."

A test of faith

Six months after her promotion, Jackie's teenage son unexpectedly died from a defective heart valve.

Despite the anguish in her grieving heart, she was able to lean on her faith and the resilience she'd developed over time. She says, "The three-and-a-half years after my son's transition was not only a test of my faith, but also represented my response to life in the face of my greatest fear."

She says now that she realized that, "Even though my son had transitioned, my ability to execute a high standard of excellence while navigating my grief reflected the strong work ethic I'd learned in childhood."

She realized the standards of excellence that she had been developing at work reflected the strong work ethic she'd learned in childhood: "My parents believed we should do our work in such a way that we would be proud to sign our names on it. The high-level performance I was able to demonstrate after the loss of my son was a testament to my ability to embody this state of being."

Despite her unfathomable loss, Jackie was still able to focus on developing her staff to become an award-winning team. She helped three women on her team earn promotions, as well as the entire team receiving

She decided to resign from Marriott and grant herself the freedom of learning how to process her grief in a healthy manner.

After a four-month sabbatical, Jackie took a general manager role with a Burger King franchise, and later with a Pizza Hut franchise. During this eight-year period, she worked to turnaround low performing restaurants by improving their employee morale, developing their self-leadership skills, and improving customer service, which led to increased sales and

Mary Eisenhauer

"I decided that I would no longer agree with anyone's opinion of me unless it aligned with my soul's truth."

profits for nearly all restaurants.

She also built her public speaking skills as a member of Toastmasters International. "I was developing my abilities to communicate in club meetings and when I started to host small group trainings in the evenings. These experiences helped me to hone my ability to create and facilitate training and development programs outside of my job."

When her job ended, she returned to Columbia, building experience in diverse fields and industries which she says "allows me to connect with so many different people at different levels. I mean, I had customers actually coming on their lunch breaks to talk to me about their problems. And that was one of the reasons why I began to start realizing, 'Hey, you can get paid for this'."

A legacy quest

Jackie's midlife reinvention began when she turned 60. "That reality inspired me to start looking at what it was that I truly wanted to do in the next 10 years," she says. She thought about her business and her health, considering what life might look like if she transitioned the skills she'd used in her corporate life into a business of her own. She'd never been interested in one-on-one counseling, but she felt drawn to group coaching.

The notion of creating an impact in the lives of more people inspired her legacy quest. She says, "This quest requires me to utilize all of my strengths, skills and wisdom I've learned to serve more people in diverse ways.

"I've known for some time that there is a greater expression of who I am, seeking to emerge and be expressed by me. I've been resistant to her because it requires me to be more visible. I've always been a worker bee, getting things done behind the scenes, producing results that positioned me to secure promotions."

Her transition meant she would have to step into the limelight. Her business became 'Be Uncommon with Jackie B' with Jackie front and center. The business provides personal, leadership and career development training and development to growth-minded self-starters and to organizations seeking to improve their performance results by investing in the development of their workforce to build a culture of trust, inclusion and high-performance.

Jackie says, "Everyone goes through spiritual awakenings, whether we acknowledge them or not. I believe they occur when life is asking us to stop ignoring or denying our truth, and when life is asking us to embrace more of our authentic self and power."

"This transition has really inspired me, Jackie says. "I've restructured my business, renaming it to reflect the deeper understanding that when our soul is well, we are well—and that everything that we do, when we begin to do it, comes from the inside."

Speaking more boldly

Jackie began building her online presence in 2009 and later started a podcast that brought her a wider audience, Her current focus is on training and teaching. "My intent is to be able to help people get connected to who they are, the truth of who they are—not the narratives of their parents, not the narratives of people and their family, not the narratives of society that says that we can't do certain things based on whatever criteria at the time is popular, but to truly listen."

As an author, she's published several books, including a success workbook in 2012, followed by *Lead to Succeed: Essential Habits for Emerging Leaders* (2012), *Get Unstuck Now: Changing Your Story Unleashes Your Power to Move On and Be Happy* (2014), *Find Your Brave: Embrace Fear As A Gift to Show Up, Shine and Succeed* (2018) and *The Go Be Great Blueprint: A More Mindful Way to Build Influence, Create Positive Impact and Accelerate Your Authentic Success* (2023).

"Even in my first book, I emphasized how my spiritual awakening in my 20s led to me accessing the transformational power that dwells within each of us."

"My spiritual awakening didn't take years," Jackie says. "It just happened over several months because of me speaking more boldly about the changes that have occurred in my life and in the lives of some of my my coaching clients."

The leader of her life

Jackie reflects that "the primary obstacle has been myself—it has been the resistance that I've had for not just embracing this with a childlike faith."

She says it's important that all women understand their own value. She believes it's important that every woman, no matter her age, understand that she is telling herself a story. "If the story is not inspiring and empowering the greatness within her, it's an indication she needs to embrace the inner work of healing heart wounds and reconnecting to her authentic self. She has the free will of choice. She's the source of her thoughts, emotions and behaviors. She's the leader of her life and has the power within her to transform her life to experience greater well-being and uncommon success at any age."

Self-assessment questions

Jackie suggests that women use self-assessment questions to increase self-awareness, identify areas of improvement, clarify goals, make more informed decisions, enhance self-esteem and confidence, and gain a structure to track their progress and measure their personal development and leadership over time.

She suggests these starter questions:
- How have your choices and actions impacted where you are now?
- What positive impact have you created in key areas of your life within the past three months, six months, 12 months, and 24 months?
- What impact have you had on your community and organization?
- How has the impact you've created influenced how you see yourself and your beliefs about what you are capable of?
- What choices will you make and actions you will take to step towards creating the change you desire and deserve to experience, now and in the future?

Jackie says that answering these questions will help women increase their awareness of how their choices and actions are directly impacting their lives now. She says that this knowledge can serve to ground them in the facts of their present reality while at the same time inspiring them to embrace the greater-yet-to-be that seeks to emerge and be expressed by them.

These questions aren't just for mature women. Jackie says. "Young women need to also begin to identify and be mindful of how their choices and actions, thoughts, emotions and behaviors are creating their reality. When they understand their values, unique strengths and abilities, they are more apt to seek environments that position them around people that support them and help them succeed. Staying where you're minimized or not valued is not healthy for any woman, no matter her age."

Trust your inner voice

Gratitude is one of Jackie's keystone personal traits. She is grateful that, from a young age, she has listened to her inner voice. "I trust my inner voice more than I trust anything else. I experienced resistance to becoming more visible, but I recognized that it reflected my fears and self-doubt. By grounding myself in the evidence of moments in my life that required me to face my fear in order to create a better life for my children, I have accepted the discomfort that comes with navigating uncharted territory."

She adds, "Every time I release resistance in my life, I am able to witness the evidence of more joy, more love, better relationships, more impact and more abundance.

"This evidence in my life and in the lives of those I serve continues to inspire me to embrace the greater-yet-to-be within me so that others are encouraged by journey to believe they can do the same. It is my hope for every woman reading this book that she feels inspired to embrace the greater-yet-be-within her and embark on her legacy quest, too."

Chantal Coupal

Life Beyond Your Comfort Zone

Chantal worked hard to free herself and her children from the damage caused by her abusive marriage. Now, after a series of career changes and medical challenges, she is focused on helping other women recover from trauma and abuse. Chantal lives in Ottowa, Ontario, Canada.

Chantal Coupal grew up without a model for a healthy family life. Her father was an alcoholic who died tragically at the age of 40 when he was struck by a drunk driver. Chantal was 12 at the time. "We were young, independent women," she says, "but he was verbally abusive with my mom. So, we never really healed, I guess. That portion of our lives led me to my ex-husband."

At age 20, she married a man she had met in high school. "I was very old-school," Chantal says. She planned to "put 100 percent effort

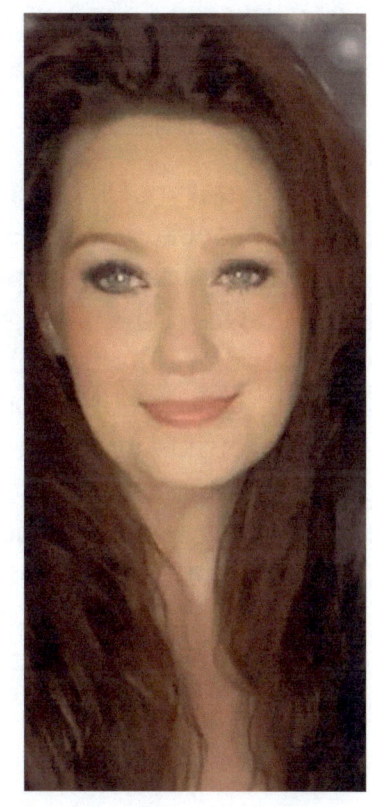

> "I think women underestimate themselves in a lot of ways. We're so strong and we've always been strong, but we don't just see it."

into that" and they were married for 22 years. She worked hard to raise their three children and have a happy family and home life. But Chantal's husband was both physically and mentally abusive. "I tried everything I could to save my marriage, to keep the peace. But in that process, I lost myself. I was always very strong and independent. I always worked. I always took care of my kids, but I was broken inside. I look back now that I've been away from it for 12 years, and I realize just how broken I was."

Healing

Separating from her husband was excruciating, as she dismantled decades of life with her husband. Once she and the children had their own place to live and the divorce moved forward, it was still challenging; no longer able to control her physically or emotionally, her husband refused to pay child support. "I had to work a few jobs, trying to keep a roof over my head. I wasn't getting any child support from him. I did not want to go to court because I had a lot of anxiety about seeing him again and dealing with the whole trauma."

Chantal found comfort and support in therapy. Her counselor helped her to build her self-esteem and encouraged her to lean into her career, surrounding herself with "good, healthy people."

Her counselor also helped her support her children emotionally. My fear was that my children would have relationships like the one I had with their dad, or that my son would act abusively toward a woman. That was what he grew up seeing from his dad. I had a lot of guilt."

In therapy, Chantal also started working on her body image. "I had gained a lot of weight throughout my marriage. I turned to food to heal my pain during that relationship."

The pain was so deep that she hit a dangerous point in her weight and overall health. So for two years, with the help of her counselor, Chantal went through the dietary and psychological process to qualify for gastric bypass surgery. "I worked really hard on getting through that and went on to have the surgery."

It has been six years since then, and she has lost 188 pounds, a tremendous accomplishment and a symbol of releasing decades of pain and struggles from childhood and her marriage with her ex-husband.

Chantal continues to work on losing the last 50 pounds but knows that after everything she has been through in life, she can do it. She still struggles with body image.

She gained back 45 pounds due to extremely low iron levels, the result of not being able to absorb vitamins properly because of the gastric bypass procedure.

"I just got to a point where I just said, 'Enough'."

Finding balance

Chantal worked in healthcare for many years, often working the night shift to work around her children's schedules. "I was always a giver," she says, "very codependent. I always gave 100 percent of myself and never expected anything in return, which was a form of abuse against myself." Ongoing sessions with her counselor helped her identify and address this tendency, which she is thankful for.

By the time the COVID-19 pandemic hit, she was "completely depleted. I was working 14, 15 hours a day and not getting paid for the extra hours." She gained back 65 pounds, partly because she had no time to think about food and just grabbed what was easiest.

"I just got to a point where I just said, 'Enough. I need a career change. I need to take care of myself physically and mentally."

Chantal's answer was to change jobs. She became supervisor of an insurance company that dealt with health benefits. "It's not a physically demanding job, and I was able to have that work/ life balance."

A shared path

Chantal's end goal was to help other women transition out of abusive relationships. "The type of counseling that I went through with my support person really helped me deal with a lot of past demons from my childhood and then also from my ex-relationship, as well."

"My end goal is to help women go through this path that I've gone through," Chantal says. "You feel like you're helpless. You feel like you can't get where you need to get, because of things that are being told to you on a day-to-day basis. That healing does not happen immediately, and so I wanted to do retreats for women that have been through the same thing as myself."

Her message? "I think women underestimate themselves in a lot of ways," Chantal says. "We're so strong and we've always been strong, but we don't just see it."

Chantal knew she didn't have the skills or finances to become a life coach right away, "so I tried to think outside the box. I reached out to some other life coaches who were already doing it, and asked if there was any way that I could just volunteer or even help support them." She offered to swap her background in marketing and event planning for experience until she can complete her training and offer retreats on her own.

Meanwhile, she works additional odd jobs, and she is learning Rakki and breath work. This learning is "continuing to heal parts of me." She also enjoys gardening and the peace it brings her.

Family dynamic

Chantal's three children are grown, but they did struggle in different ways with the aftermath of their family's abuse. Chantal says they have all worked through their past trauma, that they are all happy and successful in their lives because they were open to work through their pain. "It's been really hard for me—I don't want to be codependent with them because of my guilt of staying in that marriage. I want to be there as a mom, 100 percent, but I need to make sure to put up healthy boundaries for myself, and my children," she says.

"I'm very proud of my children," she says. "I've realized what I don't want in my life, and I've worked hard to eliminate a lot of toxic situations. I'm not scared to have a voice, which I was for so many years. I feel like now that I found my voice, I'm not afraid. It took me a long time to get to this point."

Chantal marvels at the progress she has made through therapy, intense introspection, and surrounding herself with people who support and inspire her.

A little push

Chantal understands that she is a survivor, willing to do what is needed for her own success. "You know, you have to push yourself a little bit," she says. She even ran for council in her small town of 3,000 people. She learned to speak in front of large crowds, "which really pushed me out of my comfort zone."

"I didn't get in," she says, but you know what? I got 500 votes, so I was pretty proud of myself."

She also dabbled in online dating. "I was self-conscious and so nervous—but then, I realized that I don't really need a man. I'm quite okay on my own, but it is nice to be open minded. You never know."

All of the work she has done on herself has made Chantal realize that she was always strong. "I realized that there was a lot of negative talk around me and within me, and toxic people that I allowed in my life for much too long I realized that I was always who I was inside, but I allowed fear stop me from getting where I wanted and needed to be.

"That's the biggest thing that I work on day-to-day. Don't be scared. Take a deep breath. You can do this."

Jennifer Faretra

Rescuing At-Risk Lives

Jennifer changed her lifestyle of addiction and now helps other at-risk women defy the odds and remake their lives. She lives in northern Massachusetts.

Jennifer Faretra came from a culture of poverty, crime, and partying and had bounced in and out of foster care. As the oldest of five children, she grew up plagued with uncertainty of what life would bring, but with a fierce commitment to her siblings' safety and well-being.

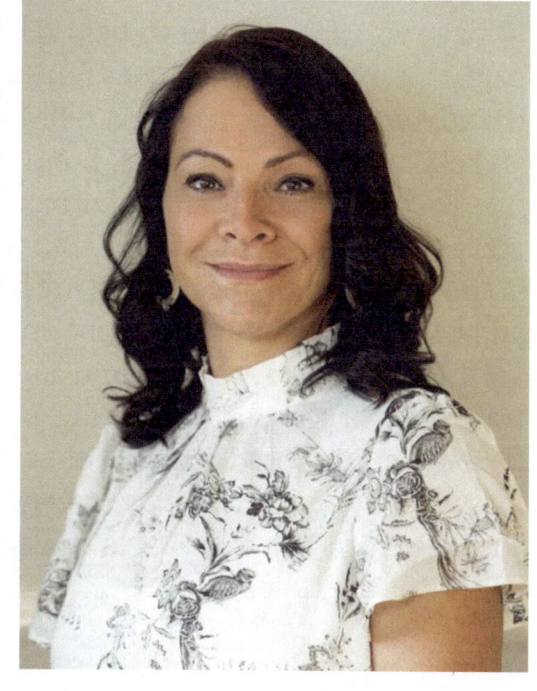

One thing that was always certain was her academic prowess. Her grades were consistently high and her teachers took notice. She showed particular promise in math in high school, which led to a scholarship for her to study engineering. She even dabbled with the idea of law school, something unheard of in her family.

College on her own

Higher education was going to be her way out of that life, she decided as she was finishing high school. Despite her rocky start in life, Jenn was going to earn a college degree and start a successful career; and she was going to be able to help her siblings be successful, too.

Jenn was a first-generation college student with no role models and no financial support, but she was determined to succeed. She found work in a group home for people with disabilities, but the pay wasn't enough to make ends meet.

"I had a good friend who was making extra money delivering drugs. I just wanted to pay my rent while I went to school. I knew it was risky and thought long and hard about helping my friend with deliveries. But the money was good and I needed to pay rent, so I started to help. The hours were flexible, I got paid a lot of money and it was fun—until it wasn't." Jenn and her friend were caught making a delivery. Her college scholarship and ability to support herself hung in the balance.

Fortunately, she emerged from that situation with monetary fines and nothing more. But six months later, she "came home from school one day and my house was torn upside down, and there was a federal warrant on my kitchen table.

"I had been so dumb, and my arrest really impacted the trajectory of the rest of my life because, at that point, I had become a convicted federal felon. And so, law school was no longer an option. There was no way I could become an attorney with a record like that. I was 19 years old and a sophomore in college at the time."

Mary Eisenhauer

"I really need to spend the next 15 years doing work that brings me joy."

She finished college at 23, graduating on the dean's list with a double major in English and psychology.

Starting over

Jenn quickly found a job in a group home for people with disabilities. She found the work to be rewarding, as she had an opportunity to help the residents see their potential and feel good about themselves. After a short time on the job, however, Jenn was not allowed to continue working there due to her felony. Unemployed, she had to figure out how to pay her bills. She found a job waiting tables and bartending and ended up staying in that work for 10 years.

In the mid-2000s, Jenn was in her early 30s and still working in bars. She worked several nights a week, making big money in tips that paid her rent and provided unlimited social opportunities, with so many types of people in and out each night.

The money she made and exposure to so many people in bars eventually led her down the path of substance use. "It was so much fun," she says. "I met so many great people, partied all the time, and made a lot of money."

Yet, on some level, Jenn knew that there was no future for her in that work. Even in the throes of heavy substance use, she knew she wanted more, and that she was capable of more.

Her wake-up call came when she found herself pregnant

with her daughter. "My life was relatively dark," she says. "I was not engaging in a lifestyle that I would want my baby to be subjected to, and I knew at that point that I had to make some decisions. I changed everything."

She walked away from that lifestyle with the help of the baby's grandmother. "Think what a nightmare that was for her. The life I was living was so foreign to her, and I was certainly not the type of girl she dreamed of for her son. She must have been horrified, but she was so good to me. She helped me stay clean and get the right prenatal care."

Taking it one day at a time, Jenn stopped using substances and gave birth to her daughter. And soon after, a son.

Claiming her reinvention

With two small children, little support from their father, and no choice but to go on public assistance, Jenn had serious decisions to make. She would qualify for subsidized childcare if she had a job. She also knew that she needed to finally finish her college degree to be able to have a meaningful career that would support her children.

There was a deadline to accept the offer of subsidized childcare, so she needed to decide quickly what her next move would be.

She was about to enter school to become a dental assistant, but fate intervened. The start date for the program was delayed by two weeks, and in that time, Jenn was offered a job as a case manager at a center for addictive behavior.

"I was so grateful for the job," Jenn says now. "I started as an entry-level case manager at $11.50 an hour and I was the only case manager on the women's detox unit. I was just so happy and grateful, you would have thought that they were paying me a million dollars a year."

Jenn dug in and built a career, finding mentors and working her way up to directing programs and facilities. At the age of 42, she earned a Master's in Social Work, enabling her to be promoted to higher-level positions at the agency, as well as supervise social work students. Her career became an example to others in the agency but perhaps more importantly, to her family.

Jenn had fought her way out of poverty, foster care, substance use, and public assistance; and worked her way into increasingly responsible roles in addiction treatment. Her own total reinvention saved her life and has enabled reinvention in the lives of others who struggle with substance use disorder.

Another turning point

After 14 years and after attaining the title of Vice President, Jenn's position at the agency was eliminated in January 2024. "I am grateful for this change," Jenn says.

"When I started this work in 2010, what I loved most about it was watching people get their lives back together. With each promotion in the agency, I found myself more and more removed from direct patient care. While I am grateful for the opportunities I have had at the organization, I have to admit, there has not been as much joy in my work over the past year.

"I have considered private practice in the past and now I am taking the leap to do it. I am opening my own practice and am getting back to my passion, which is helping people in a more direct way. I have realized that this is what fills my soul. I have had the opportunity to teach classes at the local community college over the past several years, so am also seeking to do more of that. I really enjoy teaching and am excited to do more.

"I am going to be 50 this year and I am hoping to settle into these two roles until retirement. I really need to spend the next 15 years doing work that brings me joy."

Editor's note: Jenn checked in just before this book went to press, writing: "My practice is open and thriving. I am an LLC and about to hire clinicians."

Gael Hogan

Unlimited Potential and Power

Gael Hogan has learned to use her deep spirituality to guide her career, embracing her passion for art and her work as transformational life coach, letting the power within her shape her health, relationships, and vocation. Gael lives in Fredericton, New Brunswick, Canada.

As a child, Gael Hogan could never have predicted the path her life would take. "I was kind of following a map given by my parents: 'You should be a doctor'," Gael says. "So I did the science degree."

But she soon realized that medicine wasn't the right choice for her. She worked in a lab for a few years and later at a high school.

When her first child was born, Gael realized that she

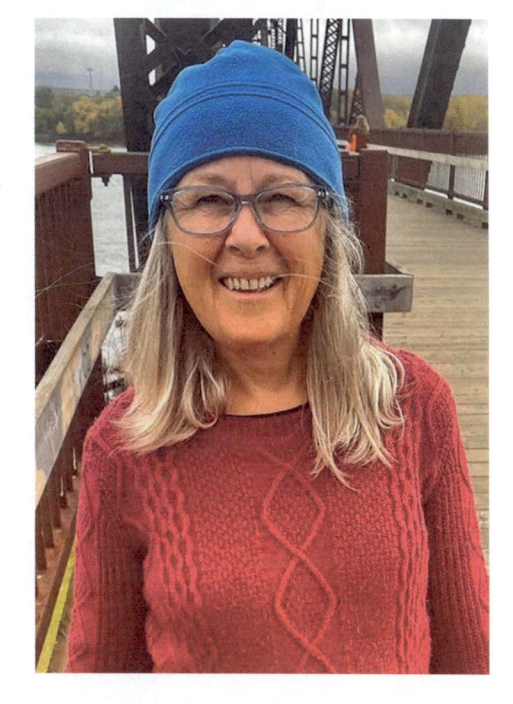

wanted to stay home and raise her family. She never returned to full-time work, but in her 30s, Gael became interested in the Spiritual Exercises of Ignatius, a set of meditations, prayers, and contemplations written by a 16th-century Roman Catholic priest, Ignatius of Loyola. 'I've always been a very spiritual person," Gael says, and her interest led to training as a spiritual director for a year-long program. "I would guide other people through their spiritual exercises journey, and that was really rewarding. I really love doing that. So, that was kind of the beginning of coaching for me."

A kind of longing

Gael loved being home with her two daughters, but when she was in her early 40s, Gael started to acknowledge "those little nigglings you get, this kind of longing or quiet whispering" to be an artist. "I just kept saying, 'No, I I'm not good enough. I can't do that. Whatever.' Then I realized that I was nurturing my children's creativity, but I wasn't nurturing my own."

Although she still had children at home—"They were always my priority"—Gael went back to university at age 41. At age 50, she graduated with the support of the artistic faculty. "They were great!" she says, joking, "I'm sure they were the only faculty at the university that didn't even notice that I was there for nine years because they are artists (themselves) and they don't care!"

What does it really mean to be happy?

By the time she finished her bachelor's degree, Gael was selling her art. "It was great," she says, "but I lost that structure of support. In my early 50s, I went through a depression after the kids left. I wasn't really making art. And so in my healing walk, that journey I went through, I started thinking about being happy. What does it really mean to be happy?"

> **"I've always been a very spiritual person... I would guide other people through their spiritual exercises journey, and that was really rewarding... So, that was kind of the beginning of coaching for me."**

She found part-time work at a Waldorf (Steiner) school, and for eight years she took care of the children after school. "I loved that," she says. "I loved children, and I was reading all kinds of books. I learned all kinds of ways of meditating. I went on a pilgrimage. I studied all kinds of things."

She realized that her painting would never take her beyond her basement studio unless she rekindled her passion for it. A 12-week life coaching course helped her bring her art back into focus, and she was soon selling at art shows.

"I thought, 'Okay, this is awesome,' and I felt like, 'I'm getting somewhere. I'm making a bit of money. This is really good.' And then I thought it would be so fun to teach other people these principles and help them get their dreams."

A difficult journey

Gael returned to the life coaching program and signed up to become a coach herself. She was excited to become provisionally certified, got her first client, and gave a couple of workshops.

But about six weeks later, Gael learned that she had breast cancer.

Gael was floored. "I was like, 'What? I finally have a direction. I'm moving. I've got energy, I've got momentum, passion—and now this. I was just flabbergasted."

Her life coaching mentor drew her attention away from the chaos that the medical issues were causing in her life by asking, "What would you love? Start focusing on what you would love, not what's happening." Her mentor refocused Gael on gratitude and growth.

"I found that hard," Gael says, "and still I'm still thinking about the gifts from all that." But she signed up for a three-day online training event that started seven days after she'd had chemotherapy.

"I did it because I was so inspired and passionate about what I was doing. I really feel that it got me through that time. I wasn't focused on my suffering. I had a better focus, and it really helped.

"That, in a nutshell, is what I've been doing. I'm finding now that, when things happen like a tree falls down, I have a perspective. There are bigger things to be upset about than a tree falling down and a fence being broken—like, nobody was hurt. There's so much to be grateful for."

A new journey

Gael completed her cancer treatments, and is getting back to her art. "It's generally been abstract, but since my cancer journey, I have been really drawn to doing chakra paintings, so I did a painting of the root chakra before Christmas and I sold it. I love that."

Gael describes her work as "a conversation between me

and the material, and sometimes something will happen that's so beautiful. I just think, 'Oh, my God.' You just get filled with this amazing joy."

She is also focused now on her passion for life coaching. "My idea was to help people my age who are looking to have more fulfillment in their lives."

She has built her practice as a transformational life coach in alignment with a commercial coaching business after completing their certification program in 2020. She now coaches clients in that method and offers workshops.

In January 2023, Gael started offering her own full-year program. "The more I work with people, the more passionate I'm getting."

"This work really is helping people to believe in themselves," Gael says. "It helps them raise their self-esteem when they say, 'Oh, I failed,' and then they can say, 'I can do this. I can learn, right? I can keep going.'"

Ellen Kaye

Embracing Change

Ellen loved being a nurse and a social worker, but the death of her husband brought her closer to her family, to new cities, and new focus on her work life. Ellen lives in South Carolina.

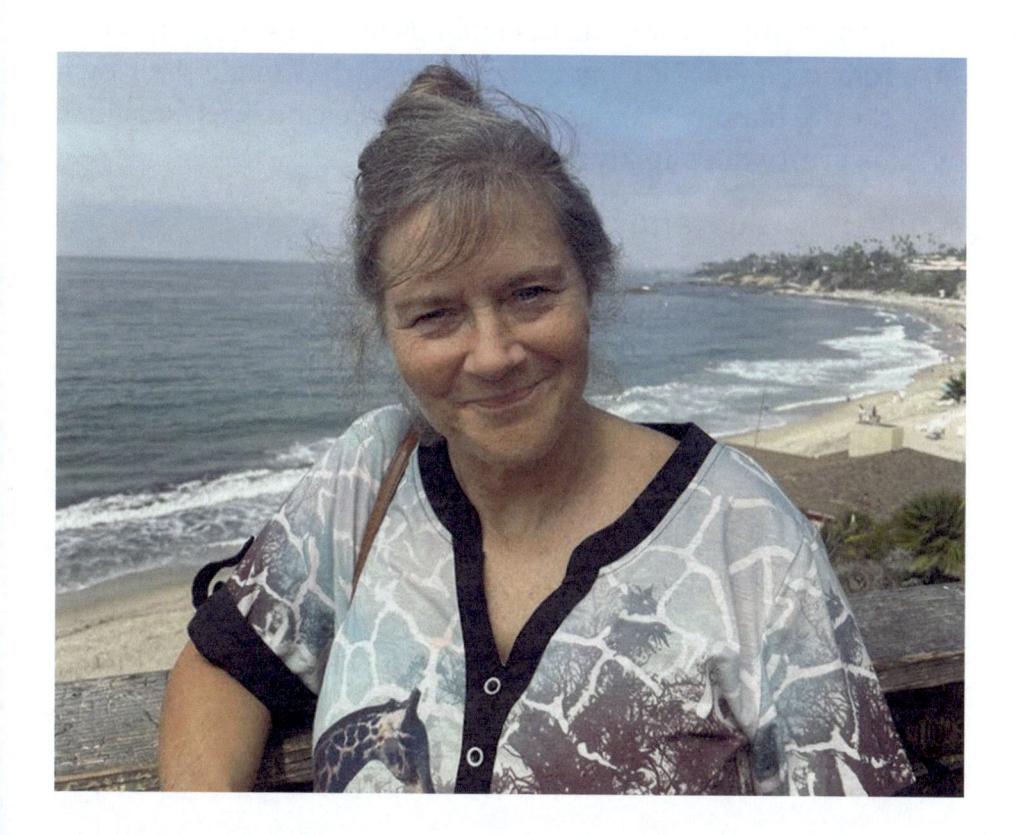

Ellen Kaye says her mother tops the list of women who inspire her. "She encouraged us to be independent. She encouraged me and my siblings to get an education and marry the people we loved but also to have a way to make our own living."

Her mother spoke from experience. Ellen's father left the family when her mother was seven months pregnant with Ellen, and then died when Ellen was only two years old. "My mother loved him very much (but) she just picked up and went on," Ellen says.

Ellen's mother brought up four children on her own. Ellen's sisters, 10 and 15 years older than she was, pitched in while their mother worked the evening shift at a Vietnam-era munitions factory. "I often say I had three mothers. At the time, I didn't like it, but now I'm very grateful because they took care of me when Mom was at work."

Ellen says that being a single mother took a toll on her mother's health, but she and her siblings prospered. "They didn't turn to bad habits, didn't get into trouble, they made their own way, they're happily married and have successful lives. Resiliency runs pretty deep in my family."

A new marriage and a career

Ellen's mother remarried when Ellen was 18. "She and I were dating at the same time," Ellen chuckles, "which was a little different." A month later, Ellen married the love of her life and they moved to Delaware. " He was my soul mate, my lifelong partner. We had rough years like everyone does, but we were always very much in love and he helped me through college. I got married in July and started at a community college in September." This whirlwind of events set the stage for the upcoming decades of change in Ellen's life.

Considering her love of animals, Ellen considered studying to become a veterinarian, but she ultimately followed her sister into nursing. She earned an associate degree in nursing and soon was working in an intensive care unit.

Over the next 30 years, Ellen and her husband moved all over the United States as she pursued her career as a travel nurse. Her various assignments brought them to Oregon, Nevada, Arizona, Florida, Montana, California, and Hawaii. They embraced the different cities, living arrangements, and people they met in every new location. Ellen's husband, a carpenter, easily found jobs with every move they made. Along the way, she realized she wanted to increase her earning power and work at higher levels.

What would you like to do?

Ellen's work in emergency rooms and the ICU showed her the connection between patient anxiety and their health outcomes. Mental health had a clear impact on patients' recovery and needed to be factored into treatment. Once she realized this connection and understood that her bachelor's degree only needed to be in a health-related field, not necessarily nursing, she asked herself "What would I like to do?"

In 2011, she completed a bachelor's degree in psychology, drawing from her love of working in the emergency room, developed a book and a program for teaching cardiac patients, and she ran a surgery center.

On the move

Ellen's many assignments brought her a wealth of experience, from developing a book and program for teaching cardiac patients to running a surgery center to working in the NICU to the emergency room. She learned so many aspects of healthcare and helped to treat patients of all ages and backgrounds. Recertification and continuing education kept her constantly in learning mode as she moved between assignments and relocated for new adventures. With Las Vegas as a home base and her husband experiencing health concerns, Ellen took travel assignments every three to six months.

"I loved travel nursing because you go in, the staff really needs help, they're excited to see you. You know they can get time off and they're glad that you're helping the other nurses to get that time. You don't deal with the politics."

Don't wait

Ellen's advice for middle-aged people: "Don't wait until you retire. Travel and enjoy your life. You never know what's next."

She and her husband enjoyed a full life. "We said we didn't have regrets. You don't know how long you have in your life. We could have saved more money. We could have had a bigger, nicer house paid off and could have had that life. But I wouldn't trade our life and our travels for anything. Those experiences were worth gold."

Moral distress

"Fast forward a few years, and now I'm getting a little older. I'm 50-something, we're living in Hawaii and I'm working 12-hour shifts. I did enjoy it. I liked my work, but was beginning to feel what they call 'moral distress'. In healthcare, we call it that because you're doing things that you can do, but not necessarily things you should do. It's a personal opinion, but it's very common in medicine." Ellen saw herself doing more for patients but in a different way, and could not envision herself doing such a physically demanding job as she reached the last decade of full-time work. There was still so much she wanted to do in her life, including more travel and spending time with her extended family, so she wanted to ease into something less physically demanding. Ellen looked back on everything she learned in her bachelor's program and on the mental health of all of her

Mary Eisenhauer

"Don't wait until you retire. Travel and enjoy your life. You never know what's next."

patients. She was still intrigued by the connection of mental health to patient outcomes, so in 2017, she took out student loans, was accepted to graduate school, and completed a master's in social work. By 2020, she accumulated 3,000 experience hours and became a licensed clinical social worker.

Change came again in 2021 when her husband unexpectedly passed away. He had struggled with health issues for the last several years and while Ellen had known time was running short, it was still a shock when it happened.

She was heartbroken. They had been married for over 40 years and had had too many adventures to count. He was her best friend and soulmate. They had traveled, moved all over the US, made countless memories, and lived life differently, together. In recent years, they had made Hawaii their home and made friends who were like family.

Ellen loved Hawaii and her community, and those friends provided unending support in the days and weeks following his death; but could she stay there without her beloved husband?

She quickly learned the answer to that question. She could not stay in Hawaii without him. It was time to move on. With her dogs and belongings, Ellen left the island for San Diego, California where she would work at the US Naval Hospital. In her grief, she found fulfillment in providing therapy to military personnel and veterans. "There's a tremendous need for this, and it's really rewarding to help service members continue to serve the country as well as support and stabilize their families.

New beginnings

Today, she is happily providing therapy via telehealth to active-duty military and their dependents. And she is remarried. "What I've learned from losing my first husband is to never say 'never.' I was not looking for anyone and was focused on settling in California for a while. I had been with my first husband since I graduated from high school and needed to figure out who I was without him. But then I reconnected with an old friend and here we are. I realize that I was very blessed to find love twice and never thought that would happen. I still miss my first husband, but it is wonderful to have another chance at a life with someone."

She's moved multiple times with her new husband. "I was very content in sunny San Diego, but getting married took me to Kansas City, Missouri where my husband was working at the time. That is never a place that I would've chosen to live. I had a preconceived notion that it was flat—no trees, boring—but I was pleasantly surprised. There were lots of trees, there were some lakes nearby, and it was kind of rolling hills where we lived, so I was totally wrong about it. That taught me a lesson that when you go someplace, you can always find positives. I was really glad to have that experience. And my job providing therapy through telehealth has been perfect. I get to continue doing what I love from wherever I live.

In 2023, my husband wrapped up his job in Kansas City. That door closed and another one opened, and we're in South Carolina. Living here has led to an unexpected joy of living near my oldest sister. I'm very happy to be near family again and my husband is near his family, as well, so there are lots of good things happening—and some lessons that I needed to be reminded of."

Veronica Robles

The Power of the Arts

Veronica moved around a lot as a child, so her roots were in music. Despite her stepfather's discouragement, she built a career as a singer-songwriter. Now, as a mentor, she uplifts other women, runs a successful cultural center, and advocates for equity in arts funding. Veronica lives in Boston, Massachusetts.

If Veronica Robles had listened to her stepfather, many lives would be very different today.

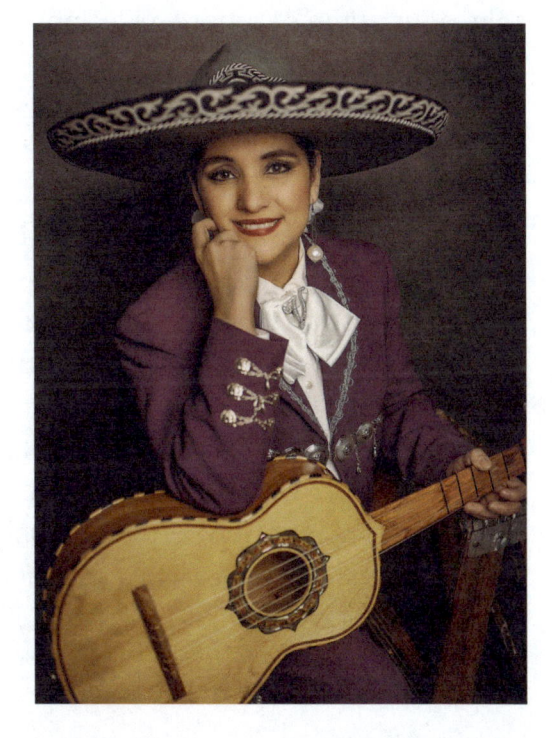

"When I was a girl, when people asked me what I wanted to be when I grew up, my answer was that I wanted to be a wise woman and sing well. I was exposed to music because my mother loved singing and my stepfather was a musician," Veronica says. "But he didn't want me to be introduced to that world because, for him, it wasn't good for women. It was a male-dominated industry. You know, too many obstacles, too many challenges, and he didn't want me to go through that difficulty. So, every time I wanted to pick up the guitar, he took it away. The piano—he took it away every time I wanted to sing."

Big extended family

Veronica grew up in Mexico, the oldest child in a family with four younger siblings, embraced by extended family nearby. "I lived a happy life with my family around the traditions that we carried," Veronica remembers. "Everybody is always dancing and singing. We joke a lot in Mexico." But, she says, she was a serious child. "I think I was too conscious about life. I think I was born like that, always hanging around adults. I was always worried about things that weren't my business."

And so, Veronica became passionate about learning from the mistakes and successes of others. "I used to embrace and take advantage of whatever opportunity was in front of me."

As a teenager, Veronica found herself drawn to performing. "I've always been social and friendly and open, and that took me to my work, which is performing and singing. I never thought that I would be a good singer. I just love singing for me. But then people noticed it, and then they started hiring me—and without me being aware of it, I was making a career."

She was successful even without formal training because she was responsible and learned quickly, so people took her seriously.

Soon, she was traveling and making enough money to help her mother provide for their household.

Veronica met her Peruvian music producer husband in New York when she was 18. They married two years later and traveled between Mexico, New York, Florida, and Massachusetts.

They settled in Boston in 2000, where they produced cultural events and Veronica performed. "I was happy because I thought that was my mission," Veronica says now. "I was bringing happiness and joy to my audiences and making people happy."

Navigating loss and illness

Veronica was immersed in singing and performing, but everything changed in 2008 when her daughter died suddenly. "She was the light of my life," Veronica says. "Kithzia was a young adult with so much life ahead of her. It was such a shock and broke my heart. It wasn't fair." At the time, Veronica describes herself as "still young and full of dreams. I didn't let anything bad affect my life. I was always positive." But her daughter's death crushed her interest in singing and performing. It was difficult to get out of bed, to find the passion to perform again.

Reimagining her life in music

Through her grief, Veronica had a different outlook and a new question. "I started thinking, 'Veronica, what is that you really want to do?' Don't think about pleasing anybody else. It doesn't matter if somebody else does or doesn't like it. It's what you want."

A few months after Kithzia's death, Veronica resumed her performance commitments. "Clients were very supportive, but I had to go back. You don't go home and stay there forever. Life goes on, and you have to somehow get back to things." She worked to find meaning in performing and to find ways to honor Kithzia.

And she received an unexpected blessing. "I always tell this story," she says, "because you never know how you will positively affect someone's life and you probably won't even know it." She booked an engagement where she was performing for more than 500 schoolchildren, teaching them to sing, and calling volunteers onstage. After the show, a teacher asked to bring a six-year-old backstage to meet her. The teacher told her that the boy had Veronica's picture and had asked every day when she would come to his school.

"He is going through a difficult time at home," the teacher told her, "but just the fact that you chose him to be on stage with you—you not only made his day, but I think he will remember this for the rest of his life." She and the teacher were emotional as they acknowledged the impact Veronica had been able to have on the boy.

Veronica realized that the music she made in the past had been about the performance; but had now become "being my true self, not only the happiness but also the sadness and the grief. And that connects me to my audiences in a very unique way."

Two years later, Veronica was diagnosed with cancer at age 38. Still reeling from her daughter's death and falling into a depression, she sought chemotherapy; but at one appointment, she says "I just didn't want it. I didn't want to fight for my life." Was it worth fighting? With such devastation over the past few years, was it worth going on? None of this made sense and none of it was fair. She found herself again struggling to get out of bed, and questioning everything around her. Why was this happening?

And then, during a chemotherapy session, she received a "dream communication," a conversation between herself and Kithzia. Kithzia's message was that, like a caterpillar, it was time for Veronica to emerge and finally spread her wings after the devastating years she'd had. "Mommy, I would never leave you because I am part of you and will always be," Kithzia said in Veronica's dream. There was a lot more life to live, and Veronica had so much more to offer the world.

Mary Eisenhauer

"I like impacting the lives of others with good messages and inspiration."

This changed everything. Veronica remembered her daughter's strength and kindness and felt supported. "Miracles happen," she says simply. And she came to a realization: "I actually didn't want to leave. I wasn't at the point that I was done with this life. I had that voice telling me, 'Let's just see the world the way it is, and let's continue working together'." She had been hurting deeply but it was time to start again.

A new way to give back

Looking back, Veronica acknowledged that it was her stepfather who had prevented her from getting a formal education in music. For a while, she considered going back to school, thinking that a degree in music could open new doors for her. After the tumultuous past few years, it was time to pursue something brand new that would bring her joy and a new direction for her life. "Then, this crazy idea came to my mind that, 'Wow, what if, instead of investing the money on going to college, I started my own organization?'"

Initially, her husband was skeptical thinking of the investments of time and money that they would need to make to get a new organization off the ground. He quickly saw the importance of Veronica's mission and "supported me all the way." She opened the Veronica Robles Cultural Center in East Boston in

2013, as she turned 40 years old. Seeing the need for such a place in her community, she says, "I was able to create an organization from nothing, without the support of any politician or any foundation, with only my family and my community."

The Center creates a space for Latinos to engage in the arts such as theater and dance, creates jobs for youths, and supports artists and other creatives. Most importantly, the Center is the first of its kind in Boston, in that it offers Latinos a space to celebrate their culture. Latino families who relocate to Boston gain access to community as well as a place to enjoy the music, dancing, and art of their culture.

Veronica also uses the center to connect the community with resources for healthcare and advocacy, something that has proven invaluable, especially in cases where English is a community member's second language.

Since the COVID-19 pandemic, Veronica has even used the center as an incubator for small businesses in the community. East Boston Chamber of Commerce, where she served as president. She was the first woman and first Latina in that role in the history of this organization.

As she has reinvented herself over the past decade, she has, perhaps unknowingly, enabled the reinvention of others in her community as they take advantage of the many resources the Veronica Robles Cultural Center provides.

Positive messages

In addition to her work at the Center, Veronica leads Boston's first all-women mariachi band and continues her music career. Performing is still Veronica's primary source of income, but the center has her heart. Her passion drives the Center to continuously evolve and offer new opportunities to the community. "I like impacting the lives of others with good messages and inspiration," she says.

Veronica rejects mainstream media and movie portrayals of Latinos as sex symbols or drug dealers. "I decided to use the power of the arts to make sure that our children and youth didn't have that idea of ourselves, and that we are more than that. Of course, we are. So, I started using this as a way for me to not only educate our own people, but other people who are not Latino so that they know our roots."

Passion Projects

The first two decades of adulthood are generally about acquiring: an education, a career, a vehicle, a professional network, a home, a partner, children. The focus is on becoming established and acquiring a particular lifestyle, especially in suburban neighborhoods where families 'keep up with the Joneses.'

Midlife presents the opportunity to shift our focus further outward, to find meaning beyond what we have already created. It is the ideal time to dabble in hobbies and special interests. Increased free time and flexibility make it easier to start a podcast or write a novel or develop a local youth group.

These projects come from a love of an idea, a childhood pastime, or even a long-lost dream. Passion projects may or may not result in income; some evolve into small businesses, while others are simply pursued for enjoyment.

The women in this section know that the key to a passion project is that it contributes to a sense of fulfillment.

Carline Bengtsson

One Experience At a Time

After a career in medical technology life sciences, Carline wrote a cookbook—and then decided to use her cooking talent to help combat hunger. Through her company Dine4Dinners®, she curates "donated dining experiences" that help fund organizations providing meals for those in need. Carline lives in Minnesota.

Carline Bengtsson used the interpersonal and management skills she developed during a long corporate career to create a retirement business based on global culinary experiences and a heart for service.

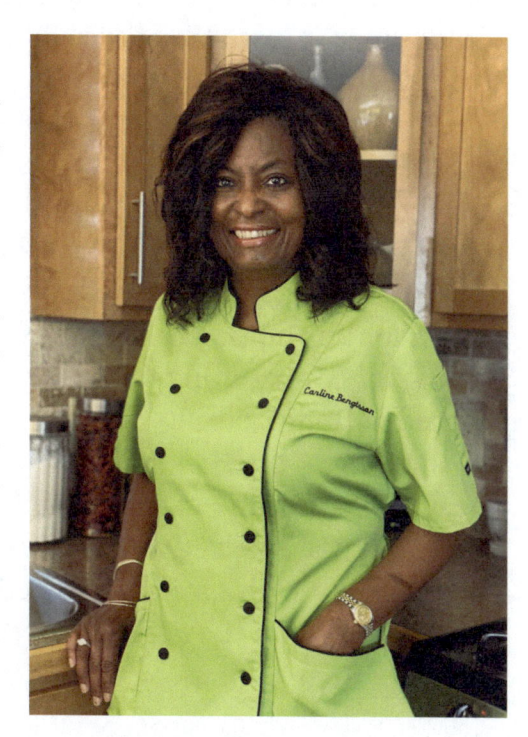

Carline was born on the island of Jamaica and immigrated with her mother to St. Paul when she was 10. Her twin siblings were born in Minnesota. Carline credits her own success and that of her brother and sister to her mother. "When you're all very accomplished, to me that says something about your family and about your mom."

She says her role models have been her mother and her counselors, teachers, and colleagues. "When you're a single parent, you get help from all sorts of other individuals—women figures in your life, you know, through your church or just within your community. And so, I learned a lot from these mother figures as well. Each played and continues to play a different role."

Stand tall

Carline says she was a shy child, "to the point that I couldn't even look someone in the eye, to tell the truth. One of those counselors—I'll never forget—put her hand under my chin, lifted up my head, and said, 'You should always look at someone when you know you're being spoken to. Stand tall.' And that was that." It was a life-changing moment for Carline, who says now: "Sometimes It just takes the right person saying the right thing to get you going in the right direction."

Carline studied art and business at Concordia University-St. Paul, which led her to work at several technology-focused corporations before she landed at medical device company Medtronic, then based in Minneapolis.

As she built a career there over more than 25 years, she felt drawn to the company's mission statement, which included the tenants of contributing to human welfare by the application of biomedical engineering and to maintain good corporate citizenship.

In 1994, Carline married the love of her life. She created a home and got involved in volunteer work. She melded her own diverse roots with his strong Swedish traditions in the recipes she offered when they entertained.

"I was seemingly moving through life, thinking this was how it was going to be until my earthly life was finished. Family and friends would always share with me openly that they thought I should open a restaurant or write a cookbook (but) these two things were literally the furthest thoughts in my mind."

But at the age of 49, Carline's life suddenly changed. In 2012, her husband died suddenly during an overseas trip. Her vision of the way life would be was shattered, as she grieved him and started to put the pieces of her life back together.

Daydreams to dinners

The following summer, she says, "I was at my desk, and I started daydreaming. I was thinking about all the comments back in the early years about opening a restaurant or writing a cookbook. And so, I sent off an e-mail to these same family and friends, asking them if they were food critics, what they would say about my cooking. There were what seemed to be immediate responses from them with incredible food reviews. And so, this was my first 'aha' moment where I thought,' Oh, my gosh, maybe I should write a cookbook'."

The result was *Carline's Fork and Cork: Simply Delish!* (CarlineB Enterprises LLC: 2015), a cookbook of fresh organic ingredients in fusion recipes incorporating flavors from Jamaica, Scandinavia, and Asia, paired with great wines in beautiful presentations. The cookbook kept her busy outside of work, a pleasant distraction to fill her free time.

As she neared her goal of working 30 years at her corporate job in the same company, her position was eliminated. Again, Carline saw life unfolding very differently than she expected, and certainly not the way she had wished for. She retired in September 2019. "I didn't have a retirement party, so to speak. I just walked out quietly, so it was truly another loss for me."

As she prepared for this early retirement, Carline redeemed her company incentive points for gifts or donations. She decided to give the points to a charity where she had volunteered. "I decided to go with that organization because in the description it said that 19 points would feed a child for 19 weeks. And right away I thought, 'employees have no idea how valuable these points are!' ...It was just such an outrageous number that I thought, 'Wow!' This was my second 'aha' moment, when I realized that what I really needed to do was to use my cooking to give back to those in need."

She was "inspired by the fact that I could use my talent of cooking and presentation of food to make the lives of others better for a day, a week, or a year." She realized that collaboration with food organizations was the key. "That have the dependable, reliable and sustainable resources to meet the needs of the hungry."

Building a following

Carline realized that the skills she had built in team and project management would carry over to running her own business. She also credits mentors and connections that she describes as meeting "people at the right time at the right moment, without even being aware." After a chance meeting with Wayne Kostroski, founder of Taste of the NFL, she sent him a copy of her cookbook and told him about her idea. The second person she told became her first customer.

"You come to find out why people are placed in your life just at the right time," she says. "All the connections I've made through my life journey at work, friendships, and several board services, elevated my cause through tangible support, which continues today."

One experience at a time

Carline launched her business website in May 2020, at the

Mary Eisenhauer

"You come to find out why people are placed in your life just at the right time."

very beginning of the COVID-19 pandemic. She offered to create gourmet meals in clients' homes. The business is for-profit, but 25 percent of the fees go to the food charity of the client's choice. "I sent out a soft launch e-mail to family, friends, and colleagues. And the next thing I knew, I had all these requests coming back for dinners." She says that the pandemic "became a positive for my business. Restaurants were shut down for several months and people wanted to continue to share in a meal around the table."

Carline expected to do an average of two events a month "so I would at least have two weekends off, but it hasn't worked out that way." She booked 19 events in the first six months.

In its first four years, Dine4Dinners® donated more than 230,000 meals, partnering with organizations in Minnesota and nationally that use dependable, reliable, and sustainable sources to provide daily nourishment to members of her community who are in need.

Carline says the business is her "baby," but she also has a team of several "ambassadors" in different roles including culinary assistants. She also gives of her time to other civic organizations such as an arts council, The Ordway, her college alumni organization including the President's Advisory Council, and the American Swedish Institute. She is a member of her hometown's Economic Development Agency.

Carline gave the commencement address at her alma mater in June 2020. "I said, as you hone your craft and follow your career path, remember: indecisiveness is not an option. Life's greatest accomplishments come from trials and failures from storms and disappointments—but most importantly, accomplishments come from every experience. One experience at a time, good or bad, catapults you, sets you up for success."

Sandy DeWeese

Helping Women Build Their Futures

Public service has always been the focus for Sandy DeWeese, but an injury took her out of firefighting and into contracting. Now, she trains other women to work in the building trades. Sandy lives in Durham, North Carolina.

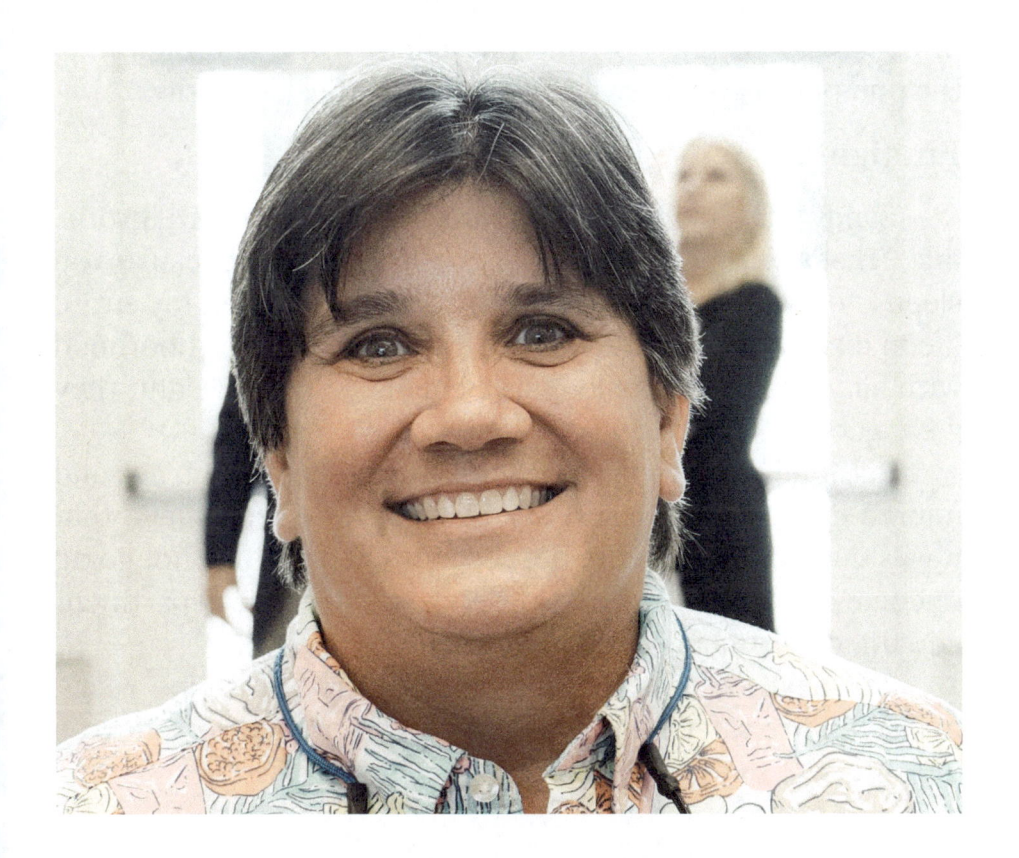

Sandy DeWeese has been drawn to public service since, as a kid, she saw the old TV show Emergency about paramedics. She applied, and was accepted. (Sandy says her mom "wasn't the happiest of mothers" out of concern for Sandy's safety, "but she got over it and was ultimately very proud of what I was.")

After trying out some entry-level civilian jobs, Sandy became a police officer in 1986 for Carrboro, N.C. Two years later, she got her chance at firefighting when she joined the public safety office in nearby Chapel Hill, doing rotating assignments: "We would spend one month in the fire department, two months in the police department, one month in the fire department."

But Chapel Hill was growing and the town eventually separated the departments. "That's a lot of continuing education," Sandy says, "trying to keep up with things in two totally different fields."

Sandy went with the fire department, realizing her dream of becoming an EMT, driving the ladder truck, and operating the pumper. "I could drive anything in the fleet," she says.

Firefighting

Sandy being in the firehouse is like having a bunch of brothers. "That's what it feels like in the fire service, because you sleep and eat together and share bunk rooms. I spent my entire life in male-dominated fields, and I grew up in a neighborhood with almost all boys. As long as I could carry my weight, they were good."

But it all came to an end when she jumped off a truck and injured her knee. "Two surgeries later, it was determined that it was time for me to retire because my knee was just not going to come back." Her total career between the police department and fire department lasted 10 years.

Her next job took her to Duke University for nine years, managing fire safety, and after finishing her bachelor's degree in criminal justice, worked in crime prevention for the campus police department.

Building a new career

Meanwhile, Sandy had helped friends do home improvement projects and discovered that she loved the hands-on work. In her mid-40s, she decided to become a general contractor. "I wanted to renovate people's houses; I didn't want to build new ones. I wanted to make people's houses better for them. So I got my associate's degree in architectural technology and, with $3,000 in my bank account, I got my license and started my construction company." Sandy formed DeWeese Construction Services in 2007.

A passion for education

A dozen years later, a chance encounter at a certification class led to a twist in the trajectory of Sandy's career when she met Nora Spencer. They talked over time, and when Spencer was ready in 2020 to begin hiring for her start-up Hope Renovations, Sandy joined the team as a trainer.

Way back in high school, Sandy had thought about becoming a teacher but her counselors had discouraged her. She'd been teaching in the architectural technology and machining programs at Durham Technical Community College, and she sponsored a $1,000 scholarship each year through the local home builders association for a woman who wanted to go to the building trades. "I decided to do was stop throwing money at it," she says, "and actually put some skin in the game."

Hope Renovations provides hands-on training for women who want to work in the building trades. The construction program provides repairs and modifications to help disabled seniors stay in their homes.

Sandy joined Hope Renovations in 2020 as a construction

"It's just really wonderful and satisfying for me when one of the trainees comes up and says, 'I made the right choice. This is where I need to be, and thank you for helping me figure that out'."

training manager and a year later became director of instruction. The COVID-19 pandemic delayed Hope's start, but 60 women graduated from the program in its first 2½ years. The students have ranged in age from 18 to 60, and with educational backgrounds from a high-school diploma to a Ph.D.

"Over the course of 12 weeks, you see them start to use the tools and things start to click—and there's aha moments," Sandy says. Along with other skills such as construction math used to build a house, trainees build small structures such as doghouses and sheds. "They truly get hands-on experience. You can hear when the hammer hits right. A couple of cohorts back, somebody's just hammering away and it hit right and that nail went in. And the trainee, just spontaneous, says, 'Man, that was sexy!'"

The program also brings general contractors, architects, and women who are already working in the industry for discussions with the students. Sandy says that it's valuable for women to see the real-world perspective. "I was never an entry-level person or just on the job site as a laborer or tradesperson so

I've never really experienced that, but some of the women that come and talk have experienced that. They share those experiences with them so that they can have an understanding of the dynamics. ...It really just depends on who you're working for, and how important it is to choose a company whose values you know match yours."

In late 2023, a year after she closed her own construction company, Sandy was named Vice President of Construction at Hope Renovations. She's found satisfaction in combining her interests in teaching and construction. "It's just really wonderful and satisfying for me when one of the trainees comes up and says, 'I made the right choice. This is where I need to be, and thank you for helping me figure that out.' It's very satisfying to know that I'm actually helping somebody improve their life."

Melissa Jenkins Mangili

Picture Perfect

Melissa's career as a neuropsychologist was fulfilling, but when her photos in an online fitness contest led to a surprise second career in modeling, she embraced it as a platform to promote positive social change. Melissa lives in Rhode Island.

A family tragedy shaped Melissa Jenkins Mangili's childhood, but she learned "how to be resourceful and to get what I needed" from her mother, who was paralyzed at age 29 in a snowmobile accident. Her father abandoned the family soon after.

"But Gardiner, Maine, is a wonderful town," Melissa says, "and if you're going to have a family tragedy, you should have it in a

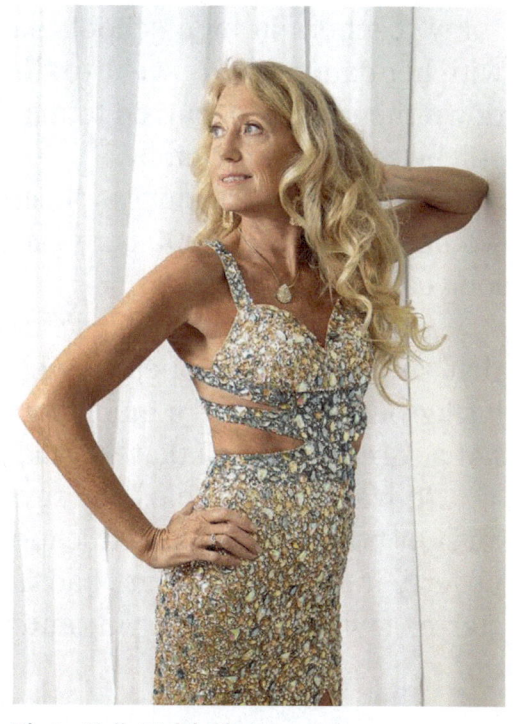

Photo: Holly Walsh Photography

town like Gardiner because everybody knows you, everybody looks out for you. So, I was raised by the whole town."

She calls her mother her role model. "She had serious health problems, but her mind was brilliant. She was so resourceful and so strong mentally. We didn't have much. We had only what we needed, so I learned from her to do what's necessary, and to prioritize things well, to structure things well—and to both give and receive help from your community."

The whole family pitched in. Melissa got a paper route at age 9 to help feed her family. As a teenager in college, she hitchhiked home so she could work weekends at McDonald's. "I had to make sure that my mother and siblings had what they needed," she says, "but also that I had a fulfilling life. I was good at school, so that became my mission."

The big gamble

"It wasn't clear to me that I was going to college, but one of my teachers in high school took me along on college tours with her daughter. We went to Colby (College), which was right down the road. It occurred to me that I could attend Colby and still be there for my family."

Melissa applied and was accepted, but had no idea how she would afford the $15,000 per year tuition. "Each year was, 'How long can I hang on?'"

As a small-town public school attendee, she also worried that she couldn't compete. "Everybody was from prep school backgrounds and had a much better education than me. It was not a sure thing at all that I would be successful."

"It was a big gamble," she says, but Melissa learned to have faith in herself, and saw education as her way out of a life of poverty in Gardiner. "I just had nothing to lose by trying. So, I started trying and kept trying and trying and trying. I didn't give up."

Finding her calling

Melissa gravitated toward psychology. "I was always an advocate," she says. "I was the one, even as a child, walking the special needs kids to class so they wouldn't be teased. With my mom being disabled and my older sister being shy, I was the one who had to speak up. I was the one who would go to teacher conferences for my little brother. I became the family spokesperson and the advocate and the listener/confidant."

Her specialty area of research was trauma. "You know, it's no surprise that I found that compelling. I had lived it."

California dreams

Melissa completed her bachelor's degree in psychology at Colby, but as she planned her graduate studies, she learned that California residents could go to state schools inexpensively. So, soon after graduation, she took a leap and "got into a Dodge Colt with 200,000 miles on it with my college boyfriend, and we drove across the country with no money whatsoever, knowing nobody in California. Not having jobs. Not having figured this out at all, other than 'We know how to work'. Looking back after all these years, Melissa chuckles at her youthful decision. But she has no regrets.

"My family laughed at me and how little I had thought through my decision. Yet somehow, we got to California." She and her boyfriend camped for the first few weeks and soon found jobs. "We stabilized. And we both ended up getting into grad school." They had established themselves.

Soon after settling in, they separated but Melissa was accepted into the doctoral program at the University of California San Diego School of Medicine. Her mother's lessons about prioritizing and about giving and receiving help served her well as she pursued her doctorate. "I somehow miraculously supported myself all along the way. I had loans, but I didn't have any family support. I didn't know anyone in California other than the people I met along the way. I just found jobs and worked my way up."

Modeling was one of those jobs. She booked department store fashion shows and other low-key gigs. "I had a neighbor who was a reporter and she would put me in her stories showing the restaurant that was popular that week, or a feature about women waiting longer to get married, and there'd be a photo of me spurning the ring. But it was like any other job to me. I never entertained the thought of doing it as a career." And she continued to focus on her studies, finishing her doctorate and looking ahead to her career.

Back to the East Coast

Melissa chose a program at Brown University to pursue her postdoctoral training, bringing her to Rhode Island where she was closer to her family. She joined the faculty after completing her postdoctoral fellowship and spent her academic career there, filling various roles as a clinical assistant professor in the university's teaching hospitals. From 1994 to 2008, she also practiced as a neuropsychologist in that healthcare system. She held the position of director of psychology for the state hospital, working with chronically hospitalized patients.

By 2009, insurance changes were forcing hospitals out of outpatient care. "So, I ended up owning my own practice," Melissa says. "It was not something I ever would have thought of doing except for the hospital pushing me out. But it was the greatest gift they could have given me because it brought me the freedom to do whatever I wanted to after that." She specialized in patients who had suffered brain injuries or were dealing with trauma or degenerative disorders, with a special interest in helping veterans.

She was at the top of her game, well-known in her field, and starting to call more of the shots in her career and life.

She started earning considerably more money in her own practice and created her own retirement plan. "I developed my independence from the university hospital. And the rest is history."

The COVID stillness

Everything changed during the COVID-19 pandemic. Even before lockdown, Melissa had worked largely from home as a consultant for doctors and lawyers. "But once the pandemic happened," she says, "there was no work. As a consultant, I met with patients in person to do assessments. Suddenly, that was no longer an option. It wasn't really a choice; I was just forced into stillness. And I started thinking. 'What's important to me? What do I really want? And do I want that life back when things resume?'"

She decided the answer was "'No'."

She wasn't sure what she did want, but she was sure she needed a change. "I felt like I was just selling my time for money. And at this point in my life, I don't need to do that. I worked so hard for my education and then for my career. I worked so hard for my freedom, so why wasn't I using it?"

An accidental reinvention

The COVID-19 lockdown was indirectly responsible for the answer to that question. "I'm a lifelong fitness enthusiast. I learned most sports as an adult, so I'm terrible at them but that never stopped me from trying. I was a runner and a triathlete. I even did the Ironman. But during COVID, we were shut down. I couldn't go to my swim team. I couldn't go to the gym or do any of the normal things I ordinarily did, and I was trying to work out alone at home, which is boring and lonely."

Melissa signed up for an online fitness group. "Some of my friends were entering a contest for 'Ms. Health and Fitness,' and that involved taking photos of yourself in workout clothes and posting them online for votes. I was just trying to find motivation during a dark time, so I entered this contest and put some photos online."

To her astonishment, she soon had more than 1,000 votes. "People liked my running selfie! I thought, 'What is up with that?' In my neuropsychology career, nobody paid attention to my important research in numbers like that." As she added more photos online, she received more and more attention. This got her thinking.

Melissa embraced the adage that, "a picture is worth way more than 1000 words. It started to occur to me that maybe, through modeling, I could develop a bigger platform and eventually use that for the greater good."

'Accidental fame'

She says that, although her Internet fame was "truly accidental, I had some inkling that I might be able to model again because I did it when I was younger." She had dabbled in social media: "I never posted many photos of myself, especially not in swimwear. I had a very conservative profile, even on Facebook."

But she created an Instagram profile and it drew attention. "It was all new to me, but I put a few self-made photos up on Instagram and photographers started contacting me, saying, 'I can take better pictures of you, and you can have them for your modeling portfolio.' We took better photos, and then I was contacted by even more photographers."

As she attracted more and more interest from photographers and social media, she also received offers to serve as an ambassador for designers, boutiques, and companies that sold workout wear. "I accepted some of the offers, and as they came

Mary Eisenhauer

"It started to occur to me that maybe, through modeling, I could develop a bigger platform and eventually use that for the greater good."

in, it occurred to me that I needed help fielding the offers. So, I started interviewing agents."

In this process, she realized that she could be an advocate for women in midlife and beyond. "There is still this unspoken bias that women over a certain age are not supposed to wear bikinis. Or if we do, we should wear very frumpy ones and be quiet—and don't take any photos because we couldn't possibly look good in them.

"There's still this real ageism. What we see in the media really does reflect our internal attitudes and our unconscious biases, and it's important to address those. Even though modeling seems like a frivolous field compared to what I've done before, it very much shapes the way that we think about ourselves."

The rest of the story

Melissa left her clinical teaching appointment at Brown in June 2021. While her practice remains open, she works only as a consultant and occasionally as a volunteer when her expertise can be put to good use.

She has also been politically active since the 2016 election, even starting a local political action group to collectively address social justice and civil rights at the local, grassroots level, and continues to work on these issues within her community. She says she is "not just an activist, but someone who actually shows up and does the work that is needed."

Her reinvention has brought her places she did not imagine at this stage in her life, including runway shows for Rhode Island, New England, and New York Fashion Weeks and in local and national ad campaigns.

She focuses on modeling, not just for the glamour but for the platform it provides her to advocate for women in midlife. And for the fun of it. "I even tried a little acting, which was so fun! I had a couple of hurdles, including a broken foot—very bad form for a runway model!—and my husband's travel bug, which kept us on the road and away from fashion events for a few months (but we had so much fun! I can't be sorry!). I'm fully recovered and back on the runway now."

Andrea Koehler

All the World's a Stage

Andrea has worked as an ESL teacher and corporate trainer, but she launched her dream career with adult coloring books with musical theater themes. Andrea lives in Seattle, Washington.

Andrea Koehler grew up surrounded by the arts. She was born in California and raised in Utah: "very white, suburban; not a very affluent home, but definitely with a lot of privilege in terms of what I had access to... My mom was a ballerina, so we grew up doing lots of what I call "Big 'C' Culture" activities: ballet, symphony, and the arts."

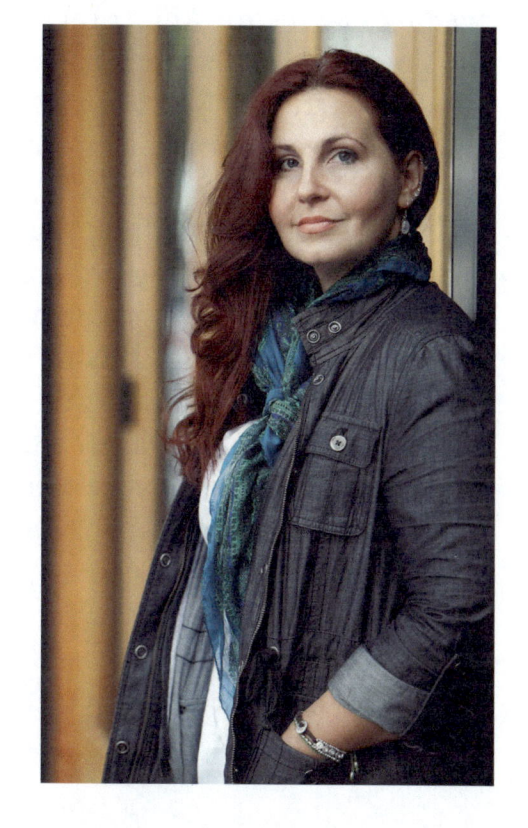

Andrea is fluent in English, Italian, and Spanish, and she wanted to travel. Her plan was to use her bachelor's degree in English literature and a master's in linguistics to fund it, teaching English overseas. But by the time she finished her degrees, she was newly married. Her husband had a business start-up in Seattle, so she ended up teaching English as a second language at the University of Washington.

Five years later, she was feeling "unimpressed" with the money she was making as a college professor—but, around that the same time, nearby Microsoft reached out to the U.W. program, saying, "Hey, we need functional business English for our non-native-English-speaking employees." Andrea became part of a team that originated a new program on Workplace English Skills, teaching Chinese-speaking employees in evening classes on the Microsoft campus.

International experiences

Andrea found her day stretched to the limits as she taught evening classes for Microsoft and then faced her own 8 a.m. class on campus. But that connection opened the door to another opportunity when she was asked to put a proposal together to create a workplace communication skills program for Microsoft in India.

Andrea taught for four years in India, and she eventually became the interim program manager, working with forty language coaches. But even though her overseas adventure ended, Andrea had a valuable takeaway. "Now I knew that there was this whole place of training and teaching in a corporate setting that paid a reasonable wage. I would not be going back to higher education." Over the next two decades, Andrea built a career as a training development manager, often working remotely from her home in Seattle.

A colorful concept

In 2015, Andrea was feeling stressed by the challenging

work environment of her then-employer, so she picked up a coloring book as a creative outlet. "Because it was the fad, right? And I spent three weeks super excited to color. And I was like, 'What is this?' ...It had the focus and the quiet and all of the nerdiness that I love so much." Andrea decided to find out what was actually going on. "My instructional design brain got working, and I started reading and doing research about the brain science behind what happens when you do creative, non-cognitive activities and you engage the three or four different parts of your brain all at the same time."

Andrea noticed that "all of the mindfulness coloring books coming out had no actual mindfulness in them. They just were a bunch of pages to color." She set out to do it better. She founded The Coloring Project in 2015 to provide "mindfulness tools for training collateral, employee and community engagement activities, and creative process building." She hosted monthly (sometimes weekly) coloring nights at a place in downtown Seattle.

The result was her book, "The Power of Positive Coloring," published in 2017.

Andrea discovered that her illustrator for that book shared her passion for musical theater. "I introduced her to 'Hamilton' and we put some 'Hamilton' quotes in a coloring page—and all of a sudden, 'Hamilton shared us' and Coloring Broadway became a thing."

She spun off the theater-focused project, and Andrea is now the Chief Coloring Officer for Coloring Broadway. "When we added coloring Broadway to the mix, it was really what brought me there was the opportunity to blend mindfulness with musical theater."

She chooses content for Coloring Broadway based on that goal. "It's a balance of what is popular and then also what shows really lend themselves to a self-awareness journey. I love it when they come in the same package; some, like 'Hadestown,' are super popular and super self-reflective."

To grow the business, she took part in theater-related maker groups and a holiday pop-up market, and started to find her market as an online shop and social media presence.

Parallel paths

Andrea continues to grow both her artistic and professional sides. In March 2020, the woman who had brought her into Microsoft and had become a good friend moved to the software development company SAP and brought Andrea on board. She took the job just as the pandemic took hold, using her free time to create content for Coloring Broadway.

But 2020 continued to be especially challenging. Her father died in August, she had a breast cancer scare in December, and in January her second husband called it quits with little warning. "Ultimately, I spent 2021 scraping myself up. I've always called it like being hit by a Mack truck, but today I was talking to somebody about it and referred to it as having a limb sliced off. It was a war wound, it was triaged and cauterized, and then I had to let that cauterized wound heal. I spent most of 2021 healing and kind of reinventing who I wanted to be now."

Andrea continues her work with Coloring Broadway and The Coloring Project. We are now shifting to include mindfulness activities in all of our materials and to retroactively fit each of our existing collections with the materials to support arts-based mindfulness activities. We're working on our first full coloring books that are driven by mindfulness activities."

Since 2020, Andrea has been a creative learning and development professional for SAP. These days, she works as an internal consultant to the executive and leadership team of the software development company SAP. "I do custom workshops for leaders and their teams, as well as doing individual coach-

"You're not late. You're not early. You get to start from wherever you're at, and it's absolutely OK."

ing." She also works externally as a coach and as a leadership development consultant."

Going back to school at some point may also be on the horizon. "With a brain that is filled with neurodivergent goodness, I am still thinking about pursuing a PhD. At this time, though, it is at least a few years out as I am looking at what else I want to do to build my career in leadership development."

Andrea continues to use her talents to support issues she cares about. She founded Any Shape or Form in 2012 "to cultivate awareness about the limiting effects of body image issues." Theater organizations are a special focus: she supports the Beltline to Broadway podcast and has also partnered with Camp Broadway and the Broadway Educational Alliance as a board member to continue arts-based mindfulness education.

Where you are

Andrea has some advice for any woman in midlife right now who is looking to make some big changes for herself. "The first piece of advice is that where you are is exactly fine. You're not late. You're not early. You get to start from wherever you're at, and it's absolutely OK.

"The second piece is it will take time. Be patient with that, because oftentimes it feels like we're running behind. I had this mental model of everything I was supposed to have at this point, but the reality is that I don't have it. I am exactly where I am, and I can't change that. All I can change is what I do moving forward."

Kyoko Nagano

Embracing and Sharing Her Culture

Kyoko embraced her own culture after a childhood abroad and has found her passion in sharing it with the world, in midlife. Kyoko lives in Kawasaki, Kanagawa, Japan.

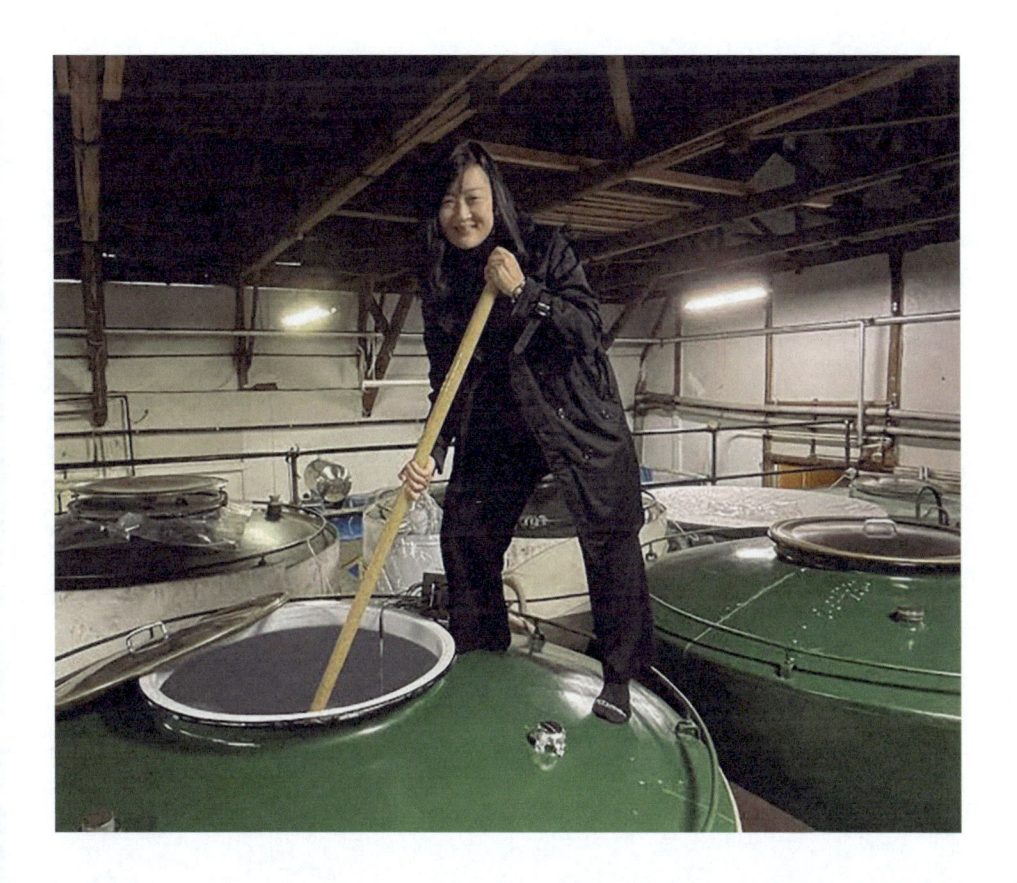

Kyoko Nagano's father worked for Mitsubishi and she grew up comfortable with the diversity of other cultures. She was born in Seoul, South Korea, and raised in Jeddah, Saudi Arabia, and the United States as the family followed her father's career around the world.

She recalls having to relearn her American accent when the family moved from Houston, Texas, to Larchmont, New York. "I had to adjust to talking the way that New Yorkers talked because everybody was telling me that I had this strong Texas accent."

Kyoko hated moving away from her friends to start over every time her father was transferred to a new job, but now is thankful for the flexibility and ability to adapt that she learned as a child. She would not have learned those valuable lessons if she had stayed in the same place throughout her formative years.

International viewpoint

She passed that attitude on to her own children as her husband took overseas posts in the United States and Thailand. "Having an international education will help them in the future, eventually," she says, adding that, unlike her own childhood, her children don't have to give up their friends when they move. "Now we're in the Internet age. You have Facebook and other social media, and you can stay connected and talk to friends. It was nothing like that when I was growing up. When I was growing up, moving meant I had to write letters to my friends (or make long-distance phone calls!) but potentially never see them again. It was much more difficult to stay in touch back then."

When Kyoko was 12 years old, the family returned to Japan to stay. Her father's travels within US-based offices were over. "I had a really big culture shock in Japan. I'm a 100% Japanese national and can speak Japanese because both of my parents are Japanese—but I was lagging behind in Japanese studies because I had been living in the United States." It took time for her to immerse herself in her native culture the same way she had been immersed in American culture for so long. But soon, she learned and came to embrace her Japanese roots.

Different dreams

Later, as an adult, Kyoko married and planned to have children. Her husband preferred that she stay at home with their two children when they were very young. "I wasn't working, because in Japan we have this proverb that if you can be with your child for the first three years after they are born, they will remember you forever." It was Japanese tradition and expectation that she not work outside the home, so she took it on.

Six years later, Kyoko re-entered the workforce. "It was not just for financial reasons (though of course, it's nice to have more money)," she says, "but I felt that I needed to go back to work to have more of a social life, rather than just meeting up with mom friends at the kindergarten. I needed to talk to adults about things other than my children. Don't get me wrong, my children are wonderful. I just needed more stimulation."

Because she was fluent in English, she found a job as an executive secretary at a large U.S.-based insurance company. She spent five years there, leveraging her bilingual skills and interacting with employees and corporate leaders from many different parts of the world. She felt fortunate to have the opportunity.

Still, Kyoko felt drawn to bigger dreams. Her elderly grandmother had told her that she had always thought there would be time later in life for travel, but she had spent her years raising children and caring for family. "My grandmother thought that she would always have time for her own dreams after she raised her kids ...But it turns out that she didn't have time." Her grandmother acknowledged the family-first tradition of Japanese culture, "but she also said that if there's something that you want to do, or if there's someplace you want to visit, you need to do it now. And then, maybe your family would understand."

Kyoko was also touched by the death of a cousin at age 44. "In his final days, he was telling me that life is too short, and he was crying. He told me that he didn't want to die. He told me that he had been so busy; there were so many things that he wanted to do in life, but he couldn't accomplish those things. He was telling me that if he had a second chance, he would love to travel or do other things he really wanted to do." She believes she was meant to hear this message from her cousin and to take it to heart.

As Kyoko's children neared adulthood, she decided that the time to pursue her own interests had finally arrived. 'It's not like I needed money to live. My husband has enough income, so it's not like I needed to work, but I wanted to work, for myself. At the same time, I felt like, 'If I can do something different and help somebody, or if I can do something that really motivates me, I think I would have a happier life."

Following her passions

Kyoko's midlife reinvention started when she decided to volunteer. She started by volunteering to help Japanese cultural teachers put on workshops with foreign nationals, drawing on her language skills. She realized that her friends in the expat community who were in Japan with their spouses were not eligible for work visas, so they had time to explore Japanese culture. She matched them with the teachers and wrote instruction manuals on where to go and what to do to learn about and experience the country. This effort took off quickly.

Mary Eisenhauer

"I feel like everybody has a different meaning of happiness. I'm happy if I can be somebody's support."

She started out volunteering on weekends while she still worked at her corporate job during the week; but her passion soon organically developed into My Pal, a service to connect Japanese artists and cultural teachers with interested foreigners through travel agencies, tourism platforms such as Airbnb, and social media. "I wanted to be like a friend introducing them: 'This is great, you should try this out'."

Kyoko found that she loved helping travelers and expats grow to appreciate Japanese culture, and enjoyed connecting them with various businesses. Over the past several years, My Pal has continued to grow in popularity as well as financially. The business works on commissions.

Through her work with My Pal, she started to think about Sake, the national drink of Japan. Travelers were typically interested in trying it, not just as a popular beverage both in the country and overseas but also because it was used for ceremonial purposes. Kyoko learned that, every year, dozens of sake breweries were going out of business. In 2018, in another effort to celebrate and raise awareness of Japanese culture, she and a friend launched Sake Lovers Inc. "to give some helping hands to the small craft breweries who need help with marketing or who don't speak English, and try to help them make their products available overseas." Sake Lovers exports to Taiwan, Hong Kong, Singapore, Canada, and Germany. "It was very much a passion project for us."

A common theme

Kyoko helped some of her brewers, artists, and teacher friends move their work online during the COVID-19 pandemic. She was the director of a marketing initiative that promoted hakko (fermented) foods before the venture folded during the pandemic. As these different initiatives come up, Kyoko finds time in her already busy schedule to give time and expertise, all to support cultural awareness.

Everything she does is connected and centered around Japanese culture. "When I came back to Japan, I wanted to introduce Japanese culture to visitors to the people who don't speak our language—to learn more about our culture."

As she describes the sake company, Kyoko explains her philosophy. "I think that if you're going after money, sometimes it drags you if you're not making a profit; but because it's my passion project, I don't get tired of working on it. People hear my stories about the sake breweries, or what kind of sake they should look into trying. I don't care if there's one person or 100 people out there. Who wants to hear from me? It's my passion."

Kyoko doesn't regret leaving her corporate career. "I feel like everybody has a different meaning of happiness. I'm happy if I can be somebody's support. If I feel like I'm supporting a talented Japanese craft artist or helping small craft sake breweries to survive, that makes my life much more meaningful."

Deborah Peel

A New Life Outdoors

Deb built her first career in corporate marketing and communications, but she left the cubicle and traditional office life behind after the COVID-19 pandemic. Now, she's outdoors, living her passion for solo hiking and inspiring others with her writing. Deb lives in Northern California.

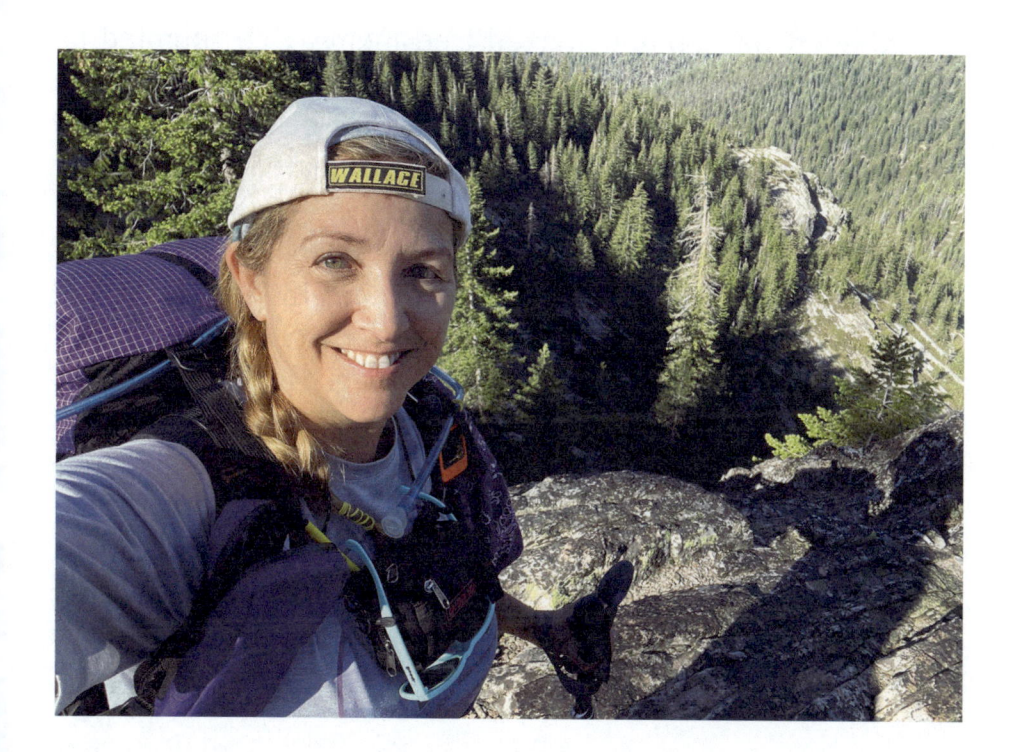

Chief Executive Hiker may be one of the coolest job titles, ever. For Deb Peel, it's also a link to her father, who literally set her on the path to her future when he introduced her to trail hiking when she was a child. Now, it describes her role in Hike for Harvey, an organization that honors her father's memory and supports Alzheimer's awareness. In 2024, Hike For Harvey's seventh annual campaign included a 75-mile hike in Scotland.

Hike for Harvey is one part of a lifestyle reinvention that she created for herself as she neared age 60.

Deb ended her 17-year career with a Northern California child services commission in 2018 as its marketing and communications coordinator. "I removed myself from the regular workplace and had to really believe in myself," she says. "I found that the hiking trail was where I was getting all my best writing and creative ideas. My creative mind was just on fire while I was out hiking."

Prepared for change

She left her job and started freelancing. Deb summed up the experience in an article for LinkedIn: "Making that change in 2018 was an incredibly scary thing to do. My heart and my head worked together to tell me it was right. I prepared by drastically reducing my debt, slashing my daily cost of living, and transitioning to a happier, simpler life. I realized that a dramatic financial adjustment was necessary to my health, happiness, and making a dream my new reality."

But her little side hustle Mountain Mojo turned into a full-on business—which was not at all what she had intended. "I ended up with a bunch of clients working my *** off, and suddenly I'm like, 'Oh my God, I've got a job!'"

Through her business and her work on Hike for Harvey, Deb realized that what she really wanted to do was to write a book. The COVID-19 pandemic changed her perspective on what was most important in her life. "I said, 'Okay, I'm going to drop most of the clients. I'm going to live really simply and see if I can make this work.' And that's what I've been doing for the last couple of years: taking care of myself and working on a book."

Ready for reinvention

Now post-divorce with grown children, Deb is on her own. "Everybody's successful out in the world, kind of doing their own thing. And I'm up here on my mountain with my dog and my cat in the house that's paid off."

Deborah says that, in her case, reinvention had a lot to do with financial preparedness. "I can't imagine the strife and the stress and the struggle of trying to keep a roof over your head when you don't know where the next paychecks come from. I absolutely simplified my life. I did it across the board financially and spiritually."

For her, it came down to the question: "'What level of survival are you willing to go to?' And for me, it's 'If I'm willing to go to the level of survival where everything I need is in a 24-pound backpack for weeks at a time, I can do this. I can pay the bills. I can figure it out.'"

Now, she says, "The distractions are gone. Spending time on the hiking trail, I become laser-focused because everything else fades away and I can really think."

On the trail

Deb spends her time on the trail enjoying nature, taking pictures, and thinking deeply on who she is and her place in the world. "I'm a real advocate for hiking and what it can do for you, mind, body, and soul. And it doesn't matter your age. I hike with people in their mid to late 70s. I hike with people in their 30s and 40s. Hiking together is a uniting experience that can transcend age, race, religion, politics. On the trail, we are simply enjoying the moment, lots of little moments."

Deb says there are multiple Pacific Crest Trail trailheads within an hour of her mountain home. As she began to hike, she met others on the trails and started chatting.

Their stories have inspired her to spend a year doing interviews that will appear in her forthcoming book, "Trail Truth," about the positive life-changing journeys of PCT hikers. "If my hikers inspire me, I know their stories are going to inspire a lot of other people," she says.

After the death of her father in 2017 and her mother four years earlier, Deb was still grieving when she took to the trail. After always struggling to feel like she belonged, her faith in brotherhood was restored by finding "the kindest people I'd ever met. I found this hiking community that was not only badass but very accepting. I really loved it. And I was talking to a lot of people, and I kept going back to the Pacific Crest Trail."

Solo hiking

One of her great joys is hiking by herself. But solo doesn't necessarily mean isolated. Since cell phones can't always connect with towers in the woods, Deb carries a satellite communication device and wears it on her pack every day. She also texts family and friends every night from camp, giving them her GPS coordinates, "just in case." "And I let them know I am safe," she says.

She also relies on "trail angels," friends, family, and even strangers who transport her to and from trailheads, and fellow hikers who support volunteering for organizations such as the Alzheimer's Association..

As a solo hiker in her sixties, Deborah says the first overnighter is "one of the scariest things a woman can do. It's a very big hurdle to get over for backpacking. I was proud to do it—but

Mary Eisenhauer

"If my hikers inspire me, I know their stories are going to inspire a lot of other people."

I wanted to turn tail and run so bad back down that trail. But I toughed it out, and from there, there was really no turning back."

One of the big lessons Deb says she's learned from hiking is the art of flexibility: "Give up the ambitious plan. See what you really need to do, regroup and turn on a dime and do it—and have a much better adventure."

For Deb, hiking is both an interior and exterior journey. Hikers stay focused, "keenly tuned for, 'What's the snap of that twig? Could there be a bear coming down the mountain?' There's things that you have to be educated in, and manage yourself out there."

At the same time, the trail provides time for what she calls her inner "trail talk." "I think that's one of the reasons that people in general, not just women, enjoy solo hiking. You can connect with others, and you can have your time alone and really grow from that."

Now, she hikes several times a week, either alone or with friends. "I get the most out of solo hiking because ultimately I find on these long trails you're really never alone. You meet people every day."

Following the path

All I can share is my experience," Deb says, "but I think the value that I have to offer to the world and the people I'm lucky enough to engage with, I think it has just intensified. I truly do feel called just to keep following this path.

"And it's so funny that my whole life has shifted to this hiking metaphor: 'If you follow your true path, and if you're brave and go around the next curve, you're going to not only have an epic view, but you're going to contribute so much more by being a happy, fully together person.

"All I can tell you is what the trail taught me. Be flexible. Be open to what comes next. It's all part of your truth."

Monica Stellmacher

Work in Progress

Monica thought she'd found her lifetime career at a phone company. But a layoff spun her in a new direction: creating an organization to help people like herself deal with the challenges of unemployment. She went back to college to become an education strategist and now pursues projects that lift up first-generation college students and the youth in her community. Monica lives in East Hartford, Connecticut.

In 2009, Monica Stellmacher got swept up in massive layoffs that followed the telecom crash. Monica had been with a "Baby Bell" phone company for 15 years–but, unlike many of her laid-off co-workers, she celebrated.

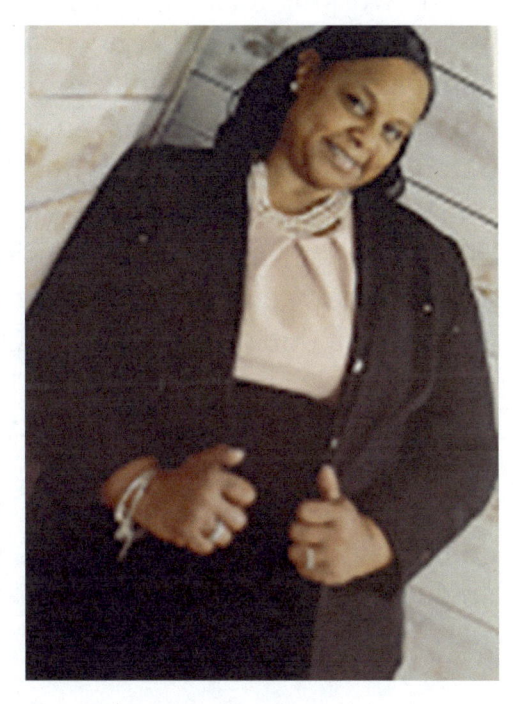

"I had been anticipating and wanting a change," Monica says. "Sometimes, if you don't move, your higher source—God, or what have you—will force you to move to the next phase. I'd probably still be sitting in that same chair if I hadn't been laid off."

Instead, with the severance package she received, she took her four kids to Disneyland. "The trip was awesome, but the layoff itself was also a blessing, the life that I needed to breathe into our family."

She needed to shake up the routine her family was living and have the time and space to consider her next move. But unlike the Super Bowl winners in a popular commercial of the time, she says, she didn't have a championship ring to pawn. "So, I took the buyout, and I started a doctorate." She was in her early 40s.

Project K.U.D.O.S.

Monica and her former phone company colleagues discovered that finding new jobs wouldn't be easy. "It was instilled in us that you get the attaché case, you put on your shiny shoes, you get the pad and pencil. And you look for a job. Well, that wasn't working for most of us."

Monica realized that it wasn't just hiring practices that had changed; it was the whole corporate model. Job search websites were different as well, and many of her former colleagues had never looked for employment on the Internet. And the 10% unemployment rate across the US in 2009 made it even more difficult for unemployed professionals to find work, much less keep up their spirits as they searched.

Having done a stint as a PTO president, Monica attended the Parent Leadership Training Institute, a program to teach the skills and tools for community advocacy. "I discovered that I had a passion to help people."

She, too, was looking for her next opportunity but felt she could help others while she did. With the right support, they could all be successful.

Mary Eisenhauer

"I had been anticipating and wanting a change. Sometimes, if you don't move, your higher source–God, or what have you–will force you to move to the next phase."

She created a group within PLTI called Project K.U.D.O.S. (Keeping the Unemployed Determined, Optimistic, and Sane). "I started holding sessions for people to talk about what it was like to be employed for a lengthy period of time with the expectation, 'I'm going to get the pen, the mug, whatever at the end. I'm going to retire from this company.' And now it was, 'Take a buyout. See you later. Good luck.' And people didn't have a clue about what that looked like. They didn't understand that, on top of looking for work and being able to support their families, there was the emotional piece of it: 'Where's my value?' 'What do I do next?'"

Monica knew how critical it was for unemployed professionals to have the emotional support of others in the same situation, along with guidance on job searching and even changing careers. The project eventually won a state citation and continues as a resource, not just for experienced workers, but for young professionals who are navigating jobs for the first time.

Monica says that the program was her transition from corporate America into the nonprofit sphere. "I think community involvement is what kept me grounded, what helped me not feel defeated in spite of being laid off. I saw a need and did what I could to meet that need."

A year of reinvention

Over the next year, Monica gave herself time to reinvent her life. "I was able to stay at home for most of the time. I threw myself into raising my family, and being a mom, and being a part of the community." She looks back fondly on that time and how it allowed her to shape her children's lives and be present for so many important milestones.

But her partner was dealing with kidney issues and waiting for a transplant. Stress caught up with Monica.

"I worked on my dissertation while he was doing dialysis. I actually got a lot done. There were nights when I was writing in the hospital while my partner slept. I was raising my kids, volunteering in the community, and being there for him at night. And nighttime seemed to be the only time for me to work on my doctorate.

"But then I had my own health issues and found myself hospitalized too. I was burning the candle at both ends and that eventually caught up with me. You can only withstand so much stress. Things will happen to make you realize it's time to reset." Her own health issues forced her to put her degree program on hold while she recovered and got her life back on track.

Graduating with her kids

Going back to college to finish her doctorate had been one more step along a winding road for Monica. She had started her academic career at Virginia State University back in the 1980s. "I joke that I discovered Virginia was for lovers, not husbands, so junior year, I had to go home—not with a degree, but with a baby, and we eventually got married."

But Monica didn't give up her goal. "I had an internal clock:

each time one of my kids graduated, I graduated. When my oldest graduated from high school, I completed my undergrad. When my twins graduated from high school, I completed my first master's. It was almost like an internal race." Not only did she delight in seeing her children succeed, she wanted to set an example of boldly pursuing her goals.

Helping first-generation students

Monica describes her college career as "a path of personal life experience, and having sat in the seat, understanding what a student and an adult in transition would need to be successful."

Throughout her own studies and volunteer work, Monica observed that first-generation students were struggling. First-generation students face unique challenges, especially impostor syndrome and concerns about fitting in, not to mention financial issues other students may not experience. Each of these factors may impact a first-generation student's success and affect the probability of the student staying in school.

Understanding the value of education in a person's life, Monica started looking for jobs that aligned her with those students.

Monica found positions at local community colleges where she quickly made a positive impact. She says she enjoys working with first-generation students and understands the challenges that nontraditional students face since she ended up having to finish her degree while she raised her own family.

She has experienced diversity efforts from both sides. "I was bussed out of Hartford to Farmington, CT so I've sat on the receiving end and have been a minority in the classroom. I know what it feels like to be the only person of color in a group on a daily basis. And I've also turned around and been able to work in another district in Connecticut with those same kids whose place I once sat in."

She has gone on to work with students from all educational and ethnic backgrounds.

Education and service

Monica continues to build on lessons she learned in childhood. Monica's father was a hospital pharmacist while her mother worked in the Hartford school system. "I had no choice but to be on the educational side," she laughs.

Monica says her parents were her role models, but her grandmother was also a big influence. "My grandmother instilled in us what we must do, being as fortunate in life as we were, and so a sense of community and caring for others fueled where I am today."

Community outreach

In conjunction with her work at community colleges and her doctoral study, Monica volunteers tirelessly in community youth programs. Again, with an eye on the importance of early intervention in children's lives and in the lives of young mothers, she lends her time to programs that focus on literacy, advocacy, and mentoring. She has even written grants to bring NASA science kits to local schools; yet another example of seeing a need and working to meet that need. She is still engaged with Girl Scouts of America, even now that her daughters are adults. She currently leads a Brownie troop and even worked for the state Girl Scout council. One Girl Scout project that has been important to her is helping to remake the Gold Award (similar to the Boy Scouts' Eagle Scout) to make its message of sustainable service more diverse to include inner-city girls.

To the finish line

These days, Monica spends part of her time caring for her aging mother but her life is still filled with academic pursuits and passionate advocacy. She is working on the final draft of her doctorate proposal and preparing for research interviews to complete her EdD degree.

As the special programs coordinator for the Elaine Marieb Adult Learner Success Center at Holyoke Community College in Holyoke, Massachusetts, she is working to launch the center's planning and logistics. The center serves adults 24 and older as well as single parents, populations she relates to and knows she will make an impact on.

"I've learned that persistence is everything," Monica says, "but persistence has to be fueled with faith, determination, and a great melting pot of relationships–support that will get you to the finish line."

Relocation and Travel

The first decades of adulthood are about becoming established. This may include buying a home with plans to stay in it for many years and spending free time renovating and maintaining the home. Having a home base creates security and comfort and facilitates routine.

Yet, leaving your home base to discover life in other places - whether short-term or long-term - often becomes intriguing in midlife. Travel is a great source of personal growth and a chance to make new memories. Having experiences in a new location teaches us about different cultures and challenges our thinking. New food, sights, and sounds enhance our creativity. Relocation can provide a new start and a shifting of priorities.

The women in this section took leaps to new places in midlife. They've found that the experience has changed them as individuals in so many positive ways.

Harumi Gondo

Accepting You for Who You Are

Harumi faced real culture shock when she went to live in Japan—but she found that conforming to those new cultural norms gave her the freedom to be herself. Now, she works to empower Japanese mothers. Harumi lives in the Greater Tokyo area.

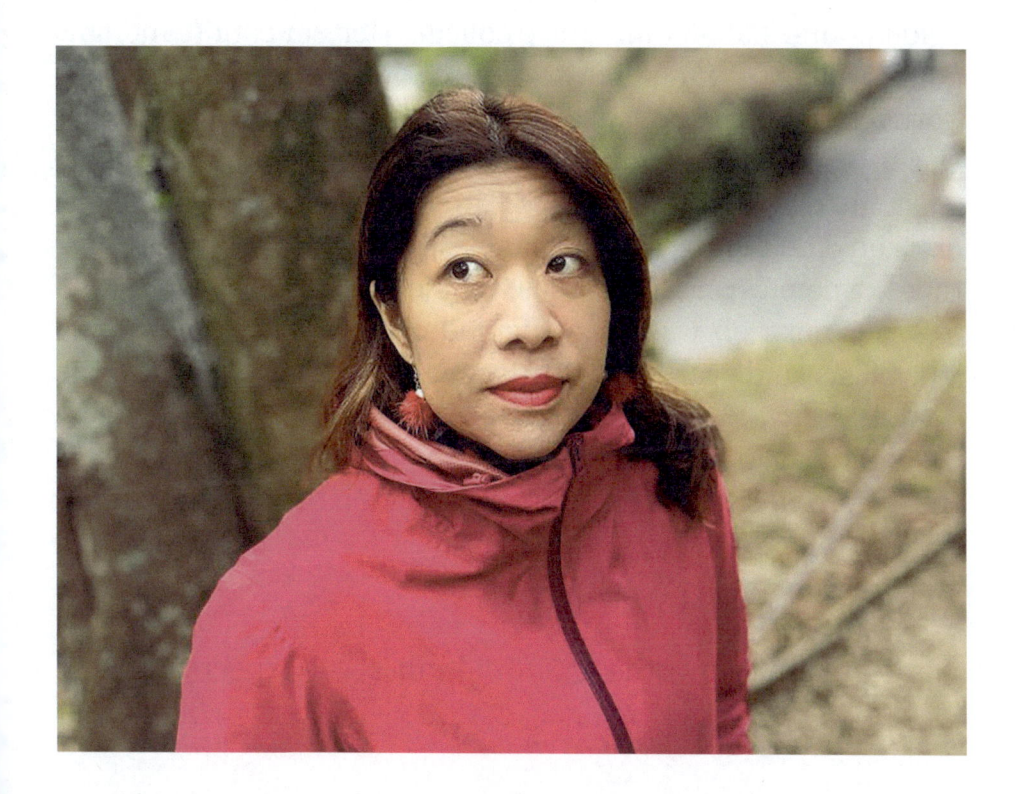

To Harumi Gondo's surprise, the strict rules of Japanese society now define her comfort zone.

Harumi was born in Japan but her parents took her to the United States when she was only 10 months old. The family moved many times to follow her father's work. "I grew up all over the country," she says. "The longest times were in Chicago and New Jersey, but I also lived in Ohio, Texas, California. Washington, DC. Boston. So many big cities. I traveled with my family a great deal."

Harumi says her parents are "totally, typically Japanese" despite the fact they lived more than half their lives in the U.S. "It's almost like they weren't really affected by their lives in America," she says. But Harumi grew up very much an American girl even becoming a U.S. citizen.

Harumi earned a B.A. in World Religions from the University of Bridgeport (CT) and her M.T.S. in Sociology of Religion from Harvard Divinity School, which enabled her to teach religion courses at a community college. Her education and language skills positioned her to be recruited to work in the New York office of a major bank, supporting their Japan Office. "That was my first experience working with Japanese people, seeing what they would do in front of Americans and other foreigners who didn't understand Japanese. I didn't enjoy being part of those dynamics and I didn't like that job."

Her next job was in media and communications, training journalists and working with journalism schools all over the world. She worked for United Press International, managing UPI's citizen journalism initiative for journalism schools and students, and later as a specialist evaluating the quality of news and feature articles.

An American point of view

"I was raised in the U.S. I did not at all expect to live in

Mary Eisenhauer

"I've created this whole life that I probably was not able to do in America."

Japan. I thought Japanese people were like nerds. In college, I did interact with some 'real' Japanese, and I felt they were repressed and in a box. And that's not how I am."

Harumi lived in the U.S. until she was 30—and then, married a Japanese man she'd met online through a close friend of her parents. "He promised to live in the U.S. but eventually found that he did not want to live there. He wanted to return to Japan. I was well aware of the gender stereotypes there and didn't want to go. I wasn't a stereotypical Japanese woman, subservient to her husband, and did not want that life. The move was a big, long discussion for us, and eventually, my husband said he was going to Japan, with or without me. It was such a hard decision; should I go with him, or stay in the US and raise my (first) daughter alone?"

Traditional Japanese men participate very little in household life. "I think that in terms of developed countries, Japan has the lowest gender equality." She says that men are often away from home, leaving the women to run the household while they are "golfing, gambling, going to restaurants with work colleagues late into the night, and leaving for work early in the morning."

Ultimately, Harumi went with her husband.

"Suddenly I found myself in Japan," she says. "And it was really not good in the beginning. It was terrible, terrible that I left my whole community in the US, my language. In the beginning, I wanted to run up to people, to tell them, 'I'm not Japanese, just to let you know.' My inner self was not Japanese."

Still, she tried to settle into the routine of daily life with her children. One day, she was visiting a bakery so small that customers walked around it in a line, and anyone who left and returned had to go through the whole line again. A misunderstanding with another woman in the line led to the woman behind her saying—in Japanese—"Just ignore her. She's a weirdo."

A splash of water

It was an epiphany for Harumi. "Weirdo" was shorthand for "hiddenness": someone on the outside. "I was like, oh, my god, I'm a weirdo, and weirdos are not accepted here. This is a country of conformity. You wear the same thing. You do the same thing. You don't say your opinion in public."

Harumi calls the realization "like a splash of water. That was a huge shock and realization for me."

Even worse, she realized, she was not conforming to Japanese society as a Japanese mom at her children's preschool. Okay, I've got to get myself in line, she thought. "In America, you do what you want. In Japan, you cannot do that. And I thought, 'My kids and I will not be accepted here unless I get my act together and conform to Japanese norms."

So, she went all in. For two years, she was quiet, observing and researching the culture. "I didn't talk much." She started conforming, and she started making friends, including an extroverted social leader who spoke a little bit of English. "We became close friends, and I would copy the things that she would wear." Harumi made it her mission to go to extended lunch meetings. "For me, it was a mission to go. I made sure I prepared conversation topics. I would talk with them. I would prepare my clothes. I was trying to copy them as much as possible—even the way I walked into the meetings."

Personality types

As a lifelong student, Harumi began studying personality type. She had always been fascinated by people's differences and interactions and found comfort in this study as she continued to acclimate to life in Japan.

This study led to an experiment: in 2013, she started TypeLAB, a mothers self-development community, which supported them to understand themselves through personality typing.

She earned a certification in MBTI, and she invited her friends to be part of her first type session. "I started conforming to the Japanese culture and that helped me to make friends, and then I invited them to be the first people in my type sessions," she says.

Personality typing sorts people by their natural preferences. The Myers-Briggs Type Indicator (MBTI), based on Jungian psychology,, groups people on four personality functions: extraversion vs. introversion, sensing vs. intuition, thinking vs. feeling, and judging vs. perceiving. From this, practitioners identify 16 personality types.

On her LinkedIn page, Harumi writes that 'identifying your Psychological Type is the first step to becoming your Ideal Self."

She started by offering the sessions for free, but quickly decided to charge for them; then steadily increased the price of her services. It was amazing to see her new community embracing psychological type. "I finally incorporated as a business and some of the women I trained are now conducting company trainings for my business, as well."

Harumi finally saw beyond the conformity. "I think through this conformity, I really disciplined myself," she says. She built her own community based on her personality types work, "and I think the beauty of a type community is we can all be ourselves."

Harumi sees her mission as more than spreading type awareness, "but to help Japanese women to build value for themselves." She officially founded a company, 16 Type, in 2022 to conduct company type trainings.

Personal growth

Harumi recalls a conversation she had with a man just before she left the U.S. to live in Japan, who told her, "Right now, it looks like it's going to be the end of the world, but you're going to come out really appreciating it." Harumi says his comment turned out to be true. "I had to train myself for myself: to become better, to be acceptable in society. But through that process, I think I also learned to understand and care for people more, so I grew as a person."

"I've created this whole life that I probably was not able to do in America," Harumi says, "but I sometimes feel like Japan is very much about conformity and not about growth." In her work both with Japanese mothers and with companies, she faces the same question: "Why do we need to grow?"

Harumi calls it "finding your life mission." "It's also about knowing your own reality, accepting you for who you are—accepting yourself."

Lisa LaHiff

A Life of Her Own

Lisa married young and joined the military a month later. She left the military to care for her disabled daughter and became a successful Realtor—only to surrender it all in an unsuccessful attempt to save her marriage. The market was crashing, so she had to start over with a new career. Now, Lisa works for the Department of Defense, forging a life of her own making. Lisa lives in Vicenza, Veneto, Italy.

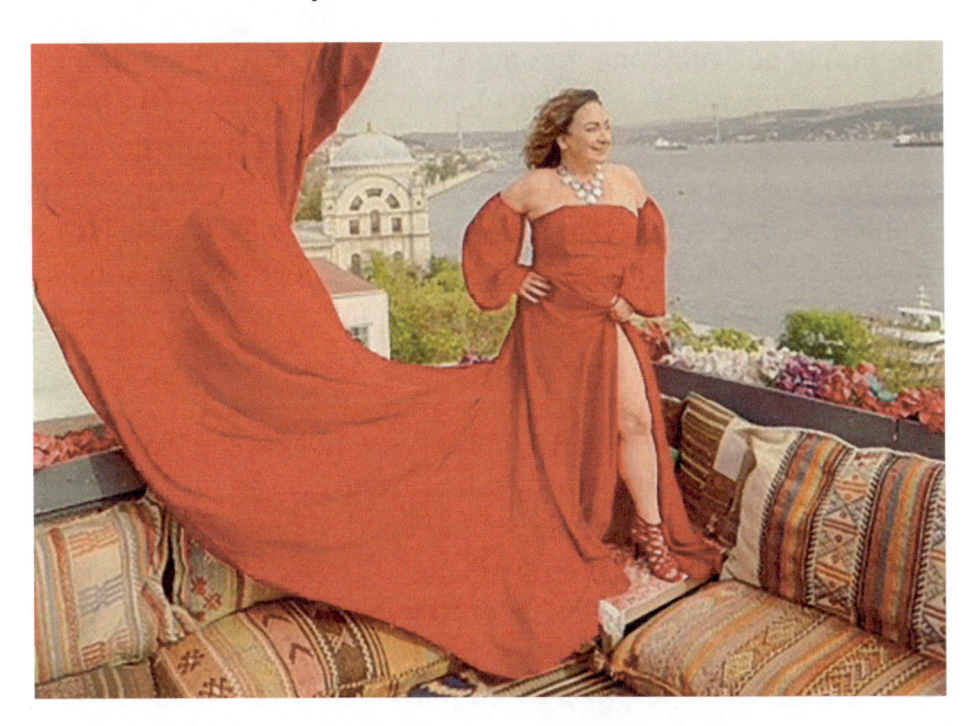

"This is no dress rehearsal. This is your one and only life," says Lisa LaHiff. She learned that lesson the hard way.

Lisa grew up in a suburb of Sacramento, CA. Her mother, who quit high school around age 14, had four children, each with a different man.

"She put two children up for adoption, she kept a third who ran away, and then had me with my father," Lisa says. "Her life plan was getting pregnant by men in hopes they would marry her, but they never did. Then along came my father. He was different. He wanted a family."

Lisa was the only one of those four children to have a relationship with her. And many, including Lisa, wondered why.

Lisa's father, a retired military man and police officer, was the only one of her children's fathers who actually married her mother. He was a college graduate, the first in his family. Lisa idolized him. "My dad was my primary parent, but he was gone all the time. He was a devout Christian—not a religious man, but a man who loved Jesus and lived the way that we should live.

Lisa's father was away from home a lot, working, because the family had only one income. "We didn't have much money, but he did charity work every chance he could and told no one, just like you're supposed to. He would save up what he could and buy coats for less fortunate kids. And so I grew up getting a philanthropic spirit. I do that myself to this day." Lisa's father was kind and warm and encouraged her in everything she did. He wanted to see her succeed in life.

A military family

In sharp contrast, Lisa's mother was not supportive, telling her that school was overrated. She saw no reason for Lisa to attend college and told her she would need to find a man because she wasn't smart enough to succeed. With this in mind, Lisa decided to drop out of high school to join the military. She chose her father's service branch to honor him, and to her amazement, achieved the second-highest score on the proficiency test.

"I thought, 'But that can't be true, because my mother's always told me I'm stupid.'"

"I got into the military and that became my plan. I was never going to have children, and I was never going to get married. I just wanted to travel the world." And she started on that path, yet still had her mother's message in her head: she was nothing without a man. She would need a man to help her succeed but she simply wasn't smart enough to do it on her own. Lisa married an enlisted Air Force serviceman.

"I went to boot camp, and they wanted me to be an air traffic controller based on my high scores on the aptitude tests. Again, I was shocked by that, and excited, but I said, 'No, if you don't send me where my husband is, I'm going to leave the military.'"

"I look back and think, 'If I had actually become an air traffic controller, that would have been an amazing career.'" But she took a job as a secretary to be near her new husband. "They sent me to Sacramento, where my husband was, and I ended up having a baby at 20 and another baby at 22. And I never went anywhere." She devoted her time to their young children and watched her dream of traveling the world slip away.

Family and college

Lisa watched her husband have the career she longed for, as he finished first an associate degree and then a bachelor's. "And then I watched him get an MBA, and it started to upset me. I had earned a GED but had never worn a cap and gown. And I really wanted that. My dad had encouraged me, and I was telling my children that they had to go to college. I wanted to set an example."

Lisa told her husband she wanted to pursue a degree, and

that it was her turn to get an education. He was not supportive, saying they could not afford it. Her mother's voice was in her head again: school was overrated and she just needed a man to support her. But a family friend encouraged her, and with the help of student loans, Lisa graduated with honors, second in her class. She had been married for 24 years and the dynamic of the marriage was slowly shifting.

"You know, when they say education is something they can't take away from you, it sounds so corny. But it's true, forever. I'm a college graduate," she says with pride.

On her own

By this point, Lisa had become a successful real estate agent. "People knew my name and they would say to my husband, 'Your wife is so successful!' But he had become accustomed to having all the glory, and he didn't appreciate my career making so much money. I think he was threatened by my success." He had risen to the rank of major in the Air Force reserves but decided to go on active duty in Pennsylvania. They would be relocating.

Lisa loved her job and the life it provided them, but loved her husband more and planned to follow him. After all, as her mother taught her, she was nothing without a man. So she quit her job and began preparing for the move. "One night I called him and said, 'I miss you so much.' He said, 'I don't want you to come to Pennsylvania. I don't love you anymore. I met somebody else.' And he cut us off financially."

Lisa says in hindsight that the failure of the marriage was "caused by both of us and our immaturities." She was shocked and heartbroken. And with no money coming in, she had to quickly figure out a plan. Their two young adult children lived with her and she couldn't restart her real estate business because the housing market had crashed. Because she had been

Mary Eisenhauer

"I've built this group of people who love me and that I love. Family isn't necessarily always blood. So, it's wonderful."

self-employed, Lisa wasn't eligible to collect unemployment. Her children's cars were repossessed from their driveway in the middle of the night, and her home was foreclosed. She moved into an apartment and shared the rent with her children. The life she had built was over and she had little to show for it.

Lisa had no choice but to file for bankruptcy. "At the court hearing, one of my creditors came in the side door and fought my bankruptcy because I'd been successful and must have had money saved. My lawyer was arguing with him and it was the darkest, most humiliating day of my life."

So she made the best of her new situation, sharing the apartment with her children and slowly making new plans. During a conversation with her (now) ex-husband, Lisa was reminded that, during her Air Force career, she had had surgery on her jaw. She was able to be classified as a disabled veteran, which put her at the top of hiring lists for federal jobs. This was a game-changer. There would be opportunities for her to rebuild her life, and she got right to work finding her first assignment.

With her adult children settled on the West Coast, she spent the next few years working in federal jobs throughout the United States. This included a position in Homeland Security in Washington, D.C., a step outside her comfort zone. But she calmed her mother's voice in her head and took the chance.

"Why wouldn't I just go for it?' she says now. "I wanted the adventure, I wanted something new. After all, I had been through, I found that I don't think like a lot of women. Particularly as we get older, a lot of women just go more and more into their little protective cocoons. I wanted to do the opposite. And I wasn't listening to the messages I had grown up hearing from my mother, anymore."

The wrong man

Lisa took another chance at dating and found a match on an online dating site. He was a massage therapist from a wealthy family who embraced her immediately. Through her new husband, she experienced the family connection she had never had in her family of origin. "His family was all from the Midwestern United States and were the nicest, most amazing people you could ever meet. I love them. They have a philanthropy group and eventually, I sat on the board. I had an incredible life with that family. I think more than I wanted to marry him, I wanted to marry them because they were such good people!" Through her connection to the family, she became a broker and reinvigorated her real estate career. Lisa felt that her life was getting back on track.

But she soon discovered that her new husband was a "narcissist abuser, and he kept escalating the abuse toward me every year we were together. He knew that, because of my Christian faith, I probably wouldn't walk away." The abuse eventually alternated between verbal and physical and put her constantly on edge. She needed to find a way out.

The final straw came after a particularly bad argument, her husband left her stranded on a country road in the dark with no way to get home. Lisa thought, "I'm 55 years old. I'm a grandmother, I served my country. I don't need this." But she went home to keep the peace and buy herself time to successfully break free from him.

"He kept unraveling more and more. I knew eventually he would kill me if I didn't get out. I put on the performance of my life in keeping him happy so that I could get my ducks in a row to leave him. I needed to go somewhere that he couldn't find me, where I would have my own money and be safe when I served him with divorce papers."

A a male therapist gave her contacts to a crisis shelter and ingrained in her: "Lisa, this is not how a man should treat you." Just as the COVID-19 pandemic hit, she rented a room in someone's garage, where she meticulously planned her divorce. Lisa eventually moved on to her own apartment in a gated community. She was free.

Lisa's Italian renaissance

Before he died, Lisa's father had made her promise that she would care for her mother in her old age. This was a big ask. Her mother had not changed a bit and was still cruel and abusive toward her. Not wanting to care for her mother but wanting to keep the promise to her father, Lisa found her an apartment nearby. She did her mother's grocery shopping and took her to lunch, but the same dynamic still existed. She didn't get any nicer with age. It was like the burden that wouldn't end."

During COVID, Lisa's mother moved into an assisted living facility. "We were still in the throes of COVID, and she was very old and she caught it. She was so frail and vulnerable at that point. The assisted living called and said to me, 'Your mom passed tonight.'

"And I just sat there. I didn't know what to say. They knew how difficult she was, how cruel she was to me. They had seen it when I visited. And they said, 'Do you want to come see her?'

I said, 'No,' and I hung up the phone. It felt like five thousand monkeys were off my back. My divorce was final a week later." Freedom had arrived. The ability to see the world and live on her own terms was right in front of her.

It was time for a change of scenery. "I had been trying to get a job in Italy for five years. I was born in Naples, Italy, when my dad was in the military and I wanted to go back I was ready for a total change." And her reinvention began.

A week after her divorce was final, Lisa was posted to Vicenza, Italy, to work as a financial analyst for the Department of Defense. She didn't know anyone in Vicenza and didn't know the language, but knew with full certainty that she would figure it all out and establish a life for herself. She quickly found a home, met English-speaking coworkers, and immersed herself in the language. "In Italy, it's not about speaking perfect Italian, it's about showing that you want to try."

In this new chapter in Italy, Lisa wanted to embrace it all. Although she hadn't driven a stick-shift car in a decade, she wanted to buy a manual transmission in Italy to prove to herself that she could. And she did. It was only a matter of time before Lisa was zipping around those roads like an Italian.

Most importantly, she formed a new circle of friends. "I've built this group of people who love me and that I love. Family isn't necessarily always blood. So, it's wonderful." Lisa was thrilled in her new environment and settled in for a great new adventure. She began to see herself retiring in Italy.

And a happy ending

When she moved there, Lisa was absolutely not looking for love. She had weathered two marriages and determined that she no longer wanted to pursue romantic relationships. She wanted to take advantage of everything Italy could offer her, she wanted to travel throughout Europe, and she wanted to continue learning the language and culture; but she saw no need to be involved with a man again.

As part of her immersion in Italian culture, Lisa decided to take dance lessons and attended a dance event on a Saturday night. "Loris (Lisa's now-partner) was taking dance lessons at the same dance school, and as soon as I walked in, I thought he was so handsome. I found myself trying to sit as close to him as possible without it being weird. Every time someone came in to sit, I moved even closer."

"We smiled at each other through the whole event. When it was over, he came up to me and shook my hand. He told me his name and I told him mine. He seemed charming. "I went up to my dance instructor and I said, 'I don't think this man speaks any English. Will you please tell him that I don't speak Italian?'

Just then Loris came up to me, kissed me on each cheek, and asked me to have coffee with him. I told him in Italian, 'No thank you, I do not speak Italian well enough." He said they could use Google Translate, but she declined.

The dance instructors told her that Loris was single. he had never married; his decades-long girlfriend had died during the COVID-19 pandemic.

"I continued to take my dance lessons. Every week my instructors would say, 'Lisa—for the love of God, please have coffee with this man. He's driving us crazy asking about you every time he comes to school."

So, I did, and we've been inseparable ever since. He even lives with me, in fact! Another thing I swore I would never do! We like so many of the same things and truly enjoy just being together. Loris really passed the test when my dog, Harley, took an immediate liking to him. They are quite a pair! We cook together, we go places, we spend time with friends. He takes care of me in ways I never experienced when I was married. And we're conquering the language barrier!"

"We both have never had what we have found with each other and we both have a deep faith in Jesus that he brought us together.

"Life is so good and I've never been happier."

Editor's note: Lisa checked in just before this book went to press, writing: "Lisa has been transferred to Germany, where she and Loris live happily with their dog Harley. They hope to buy another kind of Harley for traveling German country roads.

"At the time of this writing, Lisa and Loris plan to be married in Denmark; they look forward to eventual retirement near the ocean in Southern Italy, with land and goats and chickens and senior rescue dogs."

Lyliana Morales

Breaking All the Rules

Lyliana broke away from her strict religious family and ended up in an abusive marriage. Happiness came when she learned to care for and love herself. Lyliana lives on the New Hampshire seacoast.

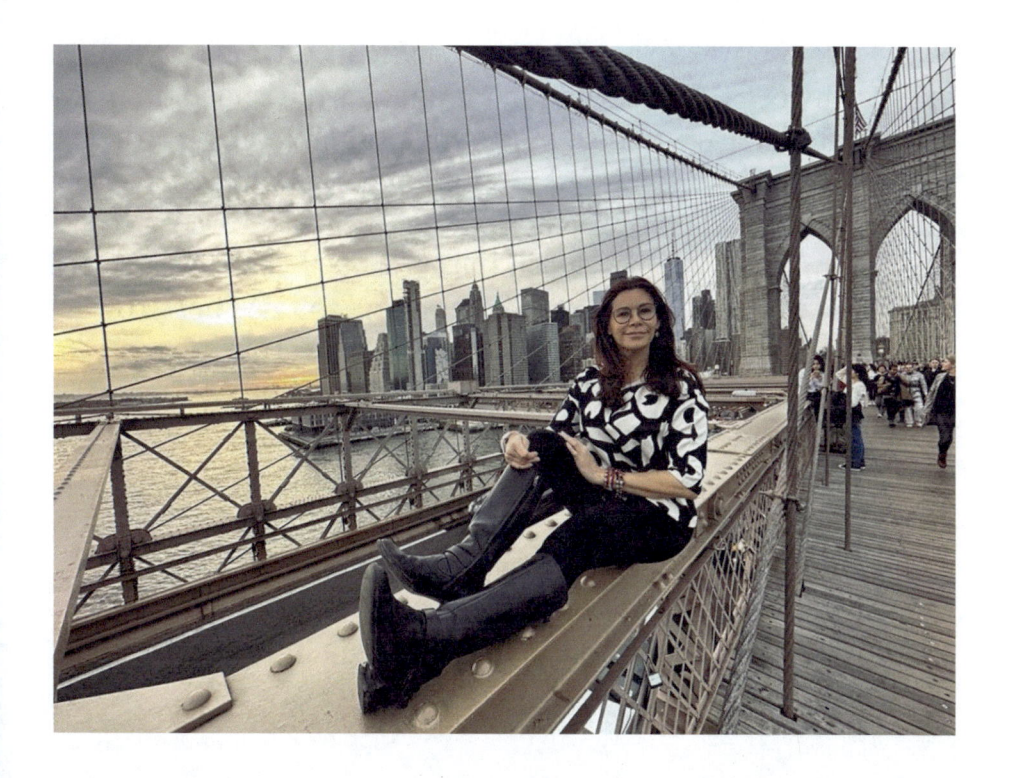

Lyliana Morales grew up in Mexico, in a strict Roman Catholic family. From the time she was six years old until age 16, Lyliana spent five hours each Saturday at meetings designed to teach her to be a "perfect housewife." The meetings, coordinated by an international conservative group within the Catholic Church on behalf of participating parishes, included lessons on cooking, problem-solving, prayer, and personal behavior. The message was: "You need to save yourself until you get married and be with your husband forever. And procreate. Kids: have tons of them."

Lyliana was assigned a personal instructor at the Saturday meetings. "She's the one who will hold your hand and take you to this world where all the girls are taught to be perfect. They teach you when to eat, how to set the table, how to make your house a home. How to say yes to your husband for whatever he wants."

A different life

"I grew up like that," Lyliana says, but in high school, "I opened my eyes. I thought about it and started questioning my mom and dad. I wanted to study something. I wanted to have a career. I definitely wanted more than what I would have as a traditional Mexican housewife."

Her mother had married at the age of 18. Lyliana was born a year later, and her mother stayed at home to raise her growing family. Her parents expected Lyliana to follow that example, to take a part-time job after high school so that she could meet a suitable husband. But Lyliana had discovered that she was good at math. "I wanted to be an engineer. I started studying and doing well in my math classes, and my parents were both really mad at me."

Against her parents' wishes, Lyliana made her own choices and completed a degree in industrial engineering. "I love that

> "It takes a lot of God's strength to let go but that strength has been there forever. ...But if you want to grow or you want to feel free? You have to learn how to let go and live. And that's not easy."

I ended up being really good at engineering," she says, "and I started living my life. I took trips, by myself, sometimes with my friends. I bought my own car. I did not wait to find a husband to buy me a car."

Along the way, she had offers of marriage, but she wasn't interested. "I don't know if that was because I was trying to have my own life, or because I wanted to go against the rules that were dictated. But I ended up having a great time with my career and my own car and my freedom!"

A troubled marriage

After years of independence, Lyliana was almost 30 when she first married. Realizing that 'her biological clock was ticking,' she settled into life as a traditional housewife and took care of her husband. "He was an excellent person," she says now, but soon they discovered that they were unable to have children. This was not the plan, Lyliana thought. She struggled to reconcile that with her early training that parenthood was her mission in life and felt a sense of failure. Her parents would be deeply disappointed. Lyliana and her husband tried fertility treatments, but the expense and discomfort of the hormones took a heavy toll on Lyliana and on their marriage.

As a final effort to help her have children and live the life they expected, her parents offered to pay for a last fertility treatment. They wanted grandchildren and believed that being a mother was Lyliana's purpose. But she had already resigned herself to the fact that it was not meant to be. If it was meant to be, it would have happened by then. "So, I started trying to find the real reason for me to be here. A different purpose. Because being a mother was not it. It took me some time to grab the whole mold and understand that I didn't fit in it. I ended up being a really good housewife, but I wasn't happy. So, I broke all the rules and got a divorce."

Another marriage, another country

"Suddenly, I felt like a wave was lifted and I felt free," Lyliana says. "I got a tattoo and then I got a second tattoo and then a third... And one of them is a set of wings because I felt that, after the divorce, suddenly I could fly wherever I wanted." Reclaiming some freedom was exhilarating. She went back to work and revived her social life.

She started dating again, reaching outside her old circles. "I felt that my home city was too small for me and I needed more. And then I met a new man who was in a different stage of life. He was also Mexican, had a great job, made lots of money, traveled the world, and had kids of his own that I could spend time with. I saw that all as an opportunity, so I got married. Which I quickly learned was a huge mistake."

Soon after they married, Lyliana's new husband transferred to a new job within his company so they relocated to New Hampshire. The company sponsored her green card so she was able to make the move as a "plus one" to her husband. This felt like a new adventure and Lyliana embraced the opportunity to start fresh, thinking they would build a great new life together. She had grown up learning English in school, which would enable her to eventually get a job and build a social circle. Once they were settled in their new home, her new life would begin.

But instead, her husband's moods became unpredictable and he was increasingly verbally abusive toward her. She found herself back in the role of housewife, in a new place without family and friends, making her vulnerable. "It was the first time that somebody yelled at me. It took strength out of me. I was constantly afraid. It was really scary, and he threatened me a lot." She started losing herself as her husband's verbal abuse became worse and worse and he threatened her green card. Lyliana became unfortunately accustomed to keeping the peace with him, to protect herself and buy time for the green card waiting period.

When that waiting period was over, Lyliana started looking for jobs, filed for divorce, and broke free.

Reinvention in America

Her parents pressured her to return to Mexico. "They told me 'You have to be either a daughter or a wife.' I was not a wife anymore because I got divorced. 'You should move back to Mexico and take care of us because it's your time to be a daughter. There's no reason for you to stay there if you're not a wife anymore.'"

But, Lyliana says, "I decided to find a job and start creating a life for me." Slowly she made friends and found a therapist who helped her, and she decided to stay in the US. It was terrifying to think about starting over, especially financially. Money had never been an issue when she was married. Her husband's income allowed her to buy new clothes for every season, take trips wherever and whenever she wanted, and join expensive gyms, not to mention cover all of her basic needs. With her dogs and a few possessions, she would be totally on her own. She was scared, but in time realized that she was surrounded by a new circle. "You realize that you have friends who really care about you. You are surrounded by people who teach you a lesson every time you talk to them. And I think that's what happened to me."

Time has passed, and Lyliana says she made the right decision. "There's a lot of reasons for me to be here. I enjoy being me, and I enjoy being where I am, and I enjoy my job. My (now) ex-husband told me I could never be successful at a job here in the US. Well, guess what? I am working in sales for a company that hired me because I'm smart and bilingual. I realize that I came to the US as a 'plus one' when I am not a plus one kind of woman. And I won't make that mistake again. I'm learning. And I've learned that I love writing. Maybe someday I'll be the one writing a book."

She stays in contact with her parents and goes home to Mexico a few times a year. Her parents haven't told their friends and neighbors about her divorce. Lyliana doesn't fit the mold of a traditional Mexican woman. But she's okay with that. "I'm not a wife and I'm not a daughter. And it feels great."

The answer in the mirror

Letting go has been a constant theme in Lyliana's life. "It takes a lot of God's strength to let go but that strength has been there forever. I had to let go of my religion and my beliefs. Sometimes I've had to let go of friends, sometimes I've let go of unhealthy situations. Sometimes I've had no choice but to let go of family members, for various reasons… And I have let go of feelings. But if you want to grow or you want to feel free? You have to learn how to let go and live. And that's not easy."

Her reinvention hasn't been simple, but Lyliana has advice for anybody considering it. "If you learn how to love yourself, it doesn't matter where you are. It doesn't matter what you do. If you're happy with yourself, you will start enjoying things you had no idea you could enjoy."

It starts with a true picture of who you are. "Open your eyes and see yourself in the mirror, and then you will know exactly what you have. You are not what you've been told. You don't have to do what society says. You just see yourself and try to get the best out of yourself.

"I started exercising again, after getting out of the habit. I really enjoy that. I started eating better. I started going to the places that I liked. I took time to go to the beach, be by myself, sit by the water, have my morning coffee alone, and enjoy my meal time. In my pajamas, if I want. I love doing that.

"Sometimes, I just leave work and go and sit by the beach and do absolutely nothing. And I owe nobody an explanation."

Joanne Robb

Travel as a Lifestyle

Joanne's business life started in retail giftware, where she owned several stores but sold them to take over her husband's financial services business when he became ill. She learned on the job and was enjoying success when the 2008 financial crisis changed things and sparked a new dream of travel as a lifestyle. Now retired, Joanne lives—among other places—in New Zealand.

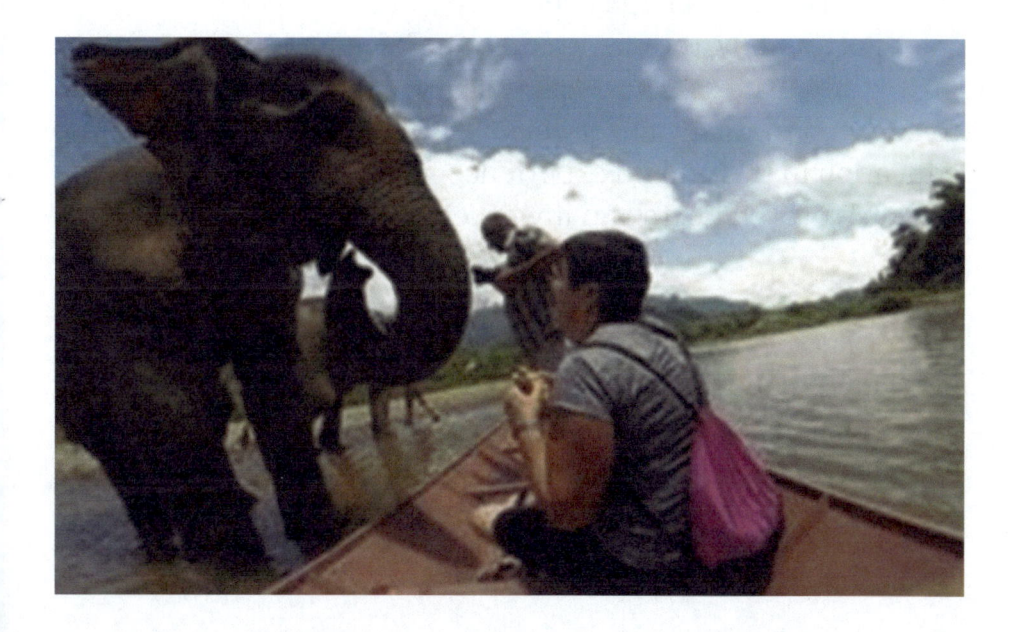

Joanne Robb left school at age 16 to work at her father's hardware store. "I quickly learned so much from him about business," she remembers. "I got very interested in the retail side of things, in all of the buying and selling and displaying of goods."

A few years later, her father leased the building next door to the store and helped her set up a small gift shop. She absorbed his interest in china, crystal, and giftware, and her father let Joanne select the stock, set up the displays, and manage the money.

By the time she was 22, she'd bought the business from her father. It was the beginning of a 20-year career in retailing, with multiple stores.

When Joanne was 35, her beloved husband fell ill—too ill to continue working, so Joanne stepped in to help run his financial services company. She was running two businesses. "It became a lot," she says, managing her own retail operation and its large staff.

Shortly thereafter, she decided to sell her own company and concentrate on her husband's business. "With no experience at all, I got thrown into the deep end of a financial services business that had a large client base," Joanne says.

"Fortunately, the clients knew me because I had been working in the business. Those clients gave me everything I needed to succeed in financial services. Bearing in mind that I had no education in this and no experience in it, I studied and had a lot of help from my peers and it worked."

Starting over

At age 38, Joanne was on her own. Her husband died, and eventually, she had to sell his business. "I had all sorts of grandiose ideas about what I would do after that, none of which actually came to fruition," she says. "I just lollygagged around for a couple of years, but none of my friends were available to play with me during the day so it wasn't as fun as I thought it would be."

After this break, she returned to what she knew: financial services. Joanne became a financial planner and built another business, doing education and financial services. "For 10 years, I actually helped people plan for retirement at the first possible opportunity with enough money to be able to live."

She was doing that same planning for herself. "I wasn't just telling people how to do it. I was walking the talk, and my goal was to walk away at some point with the option of working or not. I didn't have a particular age in mind, but I knew it would be in the 50 to 55 age bracket."

This decision was brought forward after the 2008 global financial crisis and many new regulations were put in place. "I have no problem with regulations, but they made running the financial services business very expensive and not conducive to the way I wanted to do it."

Knowing she would not be content to run it this way, Joanne brought the business into total compliance with the new regulations and then sold it. She was 50 years old.

Wanderlust

Joanne and her new partner had always taken extended winter vacations, often to the United States. "I would spend three months preparing to go away, three months away, and then three months catching up when I got back." In 2011, they spent a month in South America and then flew to Paris, where they spent two months.

That trip was the catalyst for her to want more. They had already been to Europe and done "all these crowds and all these tourists," and now it was time for a wider view. "There was so much of the world that I want to see and experience," she says.

> "I was always taught there's no such thing as can't if you want something badly enough. It might not be what you thought it might be like... But that all turned out to be fine."

"But to do it in three months every year? It was just going to take a lifetime, and I didn't want to do it when I turned 65 or older. I wanted to do it now while I was young enough to be crazy and stupid."

By Christmas 2011 she was reading travel blogs. That summer, she took three weeks off to do extensive research on how the people who wrote the blogs were traveling for $50 a day or less. She and her partner at first thought that they were not ready financially, but she started a blog of her own with the hopes that it could contribute to their cash flow. "I can do this," she thought.

It took Joanne two years to sell her business and to convince her partner that they would leave New Zealand for five to seven years. This major reinvention was underway, with no looking back. In 2014, they rented out their house (which, she says, "was extremely uncomfortable for both of us") and hit the road.

Budgeting for adventure

While Joanne enjoyed writing her blog, it did not ultimately make much of a contribution to their tight budget. They learned to make do with that budget: "If there was a choice between a taxi that was a dollar and a bus that was 15 cents? Well, guess what? We took the bus."

But they budgeted for adventure. On their trip to South America—working with a budget of $945 a week—they went back to school in Guatemala to learn to speak Spanish, swam with whale sharks in Mexico, hiked a volcano in Nicaragua to peer over the rim on their bellies to see the red lava, tried whitewater rafting in Costa Rica. Joanne's blog did afford a few perks when it brought them a complimentary day-long snorkeling trip through an underground cenote on the Yucatan Peninsula.

On the road

For Joanne, packing for these trips is an art form. "We are not as minimalistic as we would like," she says. Along with their laptop bags, "we each have a 20-kg suitcase on wheels and a 30-litre backpack each. So, we have been very lucky all around the world to each get on planes with two pieces of hand luggage."

Joanne starts planning their trips by looking at maps and making lists of the places they might like to see. She reads other bloggers she trusts who have visited those locations. Safety is always a concern, of course; Joanne learned to carry a small doorstop they could use "just in case the door lock was just not quite good enough."

They buy travel insurance but have never needed to seek major medical attention. There have been minor mishaps, such as a half-day of suffering through food poisoning, and they have sometimes passed up excursions if they looked dodgy, but, she says, "I didn't have any fear of the places we were going to."

She books accommodations in advance, finding a bed and breakfast, an extended stay with a local family, or an inexpensive apartment in the areas they travel.

Their travels have taken them to Mexico, Guatemala, Bolivia, Patagonia, the Galapagos Islands, Tibet, Nepal, China and Japan, to Cuba, to Bali, to Azerbaijan, Armenia, and Georgia. They hiked to Everest Base Camp and the Alta Via 1 in the Dolomites. And they almost made it to Antarctica, but limited funds and a head cold diverted them to Buenos Aires. "We stayed there for a month, and we just needed to decompress. When you travel around for five or six weeks. you just need to relax and be in a place where you can buy a week's worth of groceries."

Unexpected time out

In December 2019, they went home to be with family and friends in New Zealand for six months before leaving again on a trip to Bali and going on to Africa. But the COVID-19 pandemic intervened in March 2020. "I actually enjoyed lockdown," Joanne says. She made scrapbooks for their travels and volunteered for a local charity. "But I could see that we weren't going to be able to travel for a very long time. I asked my partner, 'What are we going to do? I'm not going to sit here.'"

The answer was to explore New Zealand. They ordered a new motor home and it arrived at the end of 2020. Since then, they've traveled around the country for months at a time.

For Joanne, the best part of traveling has been "the meeting of different cultures throughout the world and experiencing how other people live. It certainly has made me appreciate a lot of simple things we have."

She grew up being told "There's no such thing as *can't* if you want something badly enough. There is a way. That way might not be comfortable; it might not be what you thought it would be like. You may have to lower your expectations. That's the way it was for us, but it all turned out fine." This message—

that there is always a way—positioned her to successfully transition from her financial services career to traveling the world for now over a decade.

Joanne remembers the struggle to unwind their settled life, rent out their house, and get ready to travel. Bob Marley's song "Three Little Birds" got stuck in her head, and its message became her mantra. "I was always taught there's no such thing as *can't* if you want something badly enough. It might not be what you thought it might be like... But that all turned out to be fine."

Serial Reinvention

Some women reinvent themselves over and over, switching between a variety of careers and relocations and personal initiatives. Whether by chance or by choice, these women tend to make their marks in their chosen careers, then move on to new opportunities to have impact and connect with different people.

Variety is the spice of life, and each woman in this section can look back on the skills she has developed and the wide range of people she has met along the way of multiple midlife reinventions.

The women in this section have vastly different stories but they share strong work ethics, self-confidence, and transferable skills that serve them well wherever they go.

Molly Barker

The Art of Listening

Molly built an international nonprofit to empower young girls through running, but it was only later in life that she realized she could empower herself. She lives in Charlotte, North Carolina.

Molly Barker's leanings toward social activism started at home. Her mother was an athlete and a counselor in addiction recovery and treatment; her father was active in local Republican politics.

Molly graduated in 1982 from the University of North Carolina at Chapel Hill with a bachelor's degree in chemistry and went on to teach science and math until she completed a master's in social work.

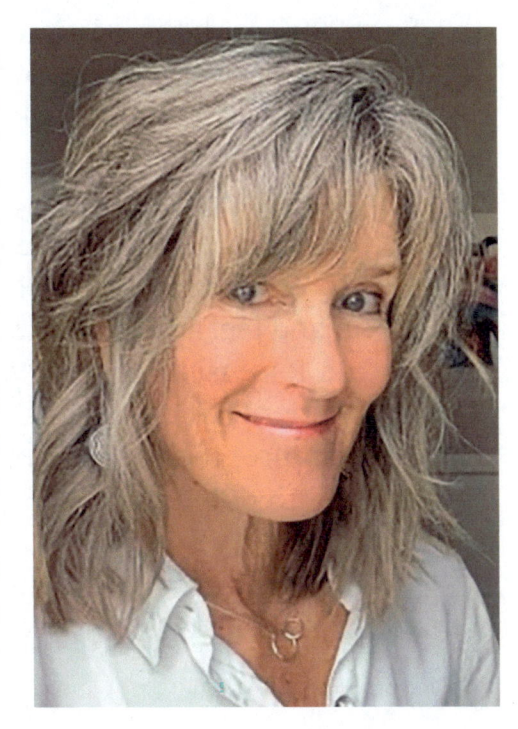

With her graduate degree, Molly worked as a social worker and counselor in the southeast United States for a few years but left the profession a few years later to train as a professional cyclist and triathlete. She credits her mother, a runner, for introducing her to running when she was a child.

Through her experiences teaching and counseling, Molly noticed gaps in school and social support for young girls. In the mid-1990s, schools were not regularly discussing issues relevant to girls, the types of issues that would shape their future success: body image, self-esteem, choosing friends, leadership, and more.

This lack of emphasis on such important topics often limited girls as they matured, Molly observed. And as an athlete, she knew the value of physical fitness and how important it was for both physical and mental health. There had to be a way she could support girls in a fun way.

Girls on the Run

So in 1996, with the mission of incorporating running into discussions of important social topics, she set up a cohort of elementary-aged girls to start Girls on the Run. She founded the program with 13 girls in Charlotte, NC, with the girls training for a 5K fun run and simultaneously learning Molly's curriculum. Looking back, Molly refers to the concept of "the girl box", defining the forced conformity adolescent girls often adopt in order to fit in and feel accepted. "The 'girl box' was an expression Girls on the Run used early on, meaning that there are these boxes that girls aren't born with. They come at us from the systems, the culture, the society around us. And we start to feel like we need to conform to those boxes. I've never been very good at that."

The nonprofit has since served more than 2.25 million girls in the third through eighth grades and has expanded throughout the US and into Canada. Each year, more than 150,000 girls participate in GOTR programs offered through more than 150+ local councils. At the end of each season, GOTR hosts one of the largest 5K series in the United States, with more than 350 events; an impressive outcome of Molly's passion for supporting girls.

In 2013, she was honored for her contributions to GOTR by Points of Light with a Daily Point of Light Award presented at a White House ceremony.

As she turned 50 and GOTR continued to evolve, Molly started to feel restless. "Not to the fault of anyone, I started to feel boxed in again. There was this desire, a sort of yearning to do something else."

While she didn't have a concrete plan for the future, Molly officially left GOTR in 2013 "I didn't really have plans for what was next," Molly says. "I just knew that I needed to go. And brilliantly, the universe, or higher power, or whatever you believe, delivered to me within weeks an opportunity to go work in Washington on Capitol Hill." And she believes that her willingness to take a risk and reinvent herself was what catapulted her into her next adventure.

Washington calls

Molly spent the next three years working with the Commission for Political Reform, a project of the Bipartisan Policy Center. "I've always been really interested in politics," she says. "It was just an amazing experience, working with a group of politicians and leaders from all over the country to determine how to improve the governing climate in Congress. I got to use a lot of material from GOTR in these discussions. But I got so frustrated with what I was seeing on Capitol Hill. I kept trying to say, 'You can change all the external rules and systems, but that does not cultivate a change in heart'." She knew she wanted to figure out how to touch people's hearts in the name of social change.

The Red Boot Way

Her time with the Commission for Political Reform led Molly to a new passion. When she left Washington, "I drove cross-country for a month and interviewed close to a hundred random strangers about what they thought was at the root of all this political divide."

She wrote up her findings as The Red Boot Way, a collection of eleven ways of interacting with people. "This change of heart, it's about deep listening, listening with curiosity and wonder, rather than judgment. It's about assuming positive intent and recognizing that every conversation matters."

Her ideas fueled the founding of another nonprofit called the Red Boot Way, based in Charlotte. "I reached out to a few people I knew professionally, and we started meeting using these steps," with facilitators who used her principles to keep the meetings on the rails. "There's a very intentional way of communicating: holding your comments to two to three minutes, and you can't cross talk, or make a statement directed at someone else."

The program took off. "We began to grow and scale that to other cities and it's still going on in some format. The material is still being used," Molly says.

She thinks The Red Boot Way was ahead of its time. "I see similar initiatives coming up now along the same lines of what we were doing." But after the 2016 US presidential election, she says, "I was being pulled into conversations where there was no movement on any topic. There was such a huge political and social divide. I just didn't want to subject myself to that over and over. You can't force people to listen."

Mary Eisenhauer

"I find great joy connecting with people during periods of transition, both theirs and mine…"

Regeneration

"This is when I went into my real unraveling," Molly says. In 2018, she retreated to Marfa, a small town in West Texas. "It's a town with maybe 1,200 people in it. It's a very artistic, very progressive little town in the middle of a huge desert with mountains. I went there and nobody knew who I was.

"It was the first time I'd ever been alone. I'd always been somebody's parent or daughter or employer or leader. But I sold everything I owned—I actually gave it away—and packed up my two dogs and went to Marfa, alone." Adopting a minimalist lifestyle and trimming her expenses, Molly stayed in Marfa until the end of 2023.

"Doing nothing was actually doing something for me," Molly says now. "I've never done 'nothing.' I had always felt this obligation to always be doing for others, always this sort of manufactured busyness, this sense of urgency. I never considered, 'What do I want or need?'"

She recalls a day after she'd been in Texas for a few months when she had nothing to do. She asked herself, "What would you like to do?' I felt like coloring. So I bought a coloring book and colored, and I watched something on Netflix, and I ate a good meal in that moment. Those were the things I wanted to do." She recognizes that this freedom was a luxury. "Not everybody has this choice."

Full circle

While in Marfa, Molly bought a bike and rediscovered being an athlete. Her competitive spirit returned and she started winning at cycling events, but with a new outlook. "I only competed when I felt like it. It was truly a luxury, and it was so beautiful. Being in a new town with the landscape, the hiking, the close friends I made; even during COVID, it was a real privilege to be in Marfa, which was relatively safe."

Molly's reinvention

Molly is back in North Carolina now. She no longer competes in elite-level triathlons and cycling events but still loves to ride her bike for fun. "I am doing a few short triathlons. I run with my dog, but it's mostly in the woods and there's no goal to it. I'm running for myself and it feels good."

She has also made peace with getting older: "You know, about how aging and how my body looks and how my skin looks. I've just released all that. It distracts us, right? It's the thing that keeps us from addressing the unsettledness."

Molly has built a reputation as a motivational speaker, which has been a rewarding way of supporting herself. 'I continue to do a lot of public speaking. It's something I absolutely love to do. I speak to nonprofits and center much of what I say around the work of GOTR and the Red Boot Way. One of the best parts is that I've started driving to speaking engagements no matter how far away they are, so I can bring my dogs and camp along the way. I stay in Airbnbs where I can cook my own food. It's a simpler lifestyle than I used to have. There's no sense of urgency and I love it."

Her LinkedIn profile sums up her life's work and ongoing reinvention. It says "I find great joy connecting with people during periods of transition, both theirs and mine, and hope that whatever I do in this world challenges individuals and organizations to step outside their comfort zones and into their highest potential. I am a minimalist, unconventional in my approach toward most things, including how I live my life. I do a lot of work in the affordable housing realm and speak out and up on issues related to race and gender."

Molly is hoping to set an example for her grown daughter and other women to live their lives outside of the 'box.' "I would love for them to always find a way, no matter what season of life they're in, to put themselves first sometimes. When you have young children, it's hard to do that. But I'm hoping that I set enough of an example that they see that, and that just becomes a normal way of being."

Ann Bordeleau

Go With What Resonates

Ann, formerly a corporate travel specialist, is now a licensed massage therapist, Reiki Master Teacher, and Energy Clearer. She lives in New Hampshire.

Ann Bordeleau is an alternative medicine practitioner and energy healer, working to help clients explore their inner journeys. But long before her career move, Ann was focused on journeys of her own.

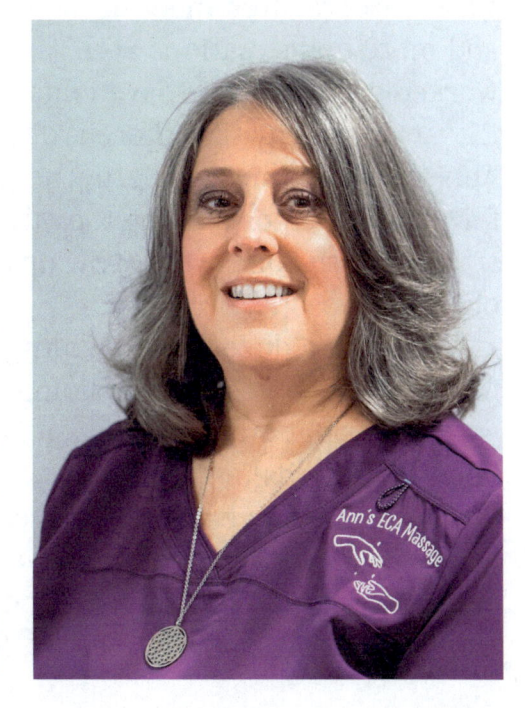

Ann's life in Nashua, New Hampshire, started with her feet firmly on the ground. Her early education was in small Catholic schools, but she transferred in 10th grade to a co-ed public high school with several thousand students. "It was complete culture shock–from the number of kids there to the entire curriculum," she says.

During her senior year of high school, Ann found a job as a data operator at a bank and considered taking evening classes at the local college. But as she researched classes, she came across information about a travel school in Kissimmee, Florida. "It was something that really piqued my interest," Ann says. "Growing up, I had wanted to be a flight attendant. I had always had this feeling of not wanting to stay in Nashua; there was nothing for me in Nashua."

Taking flight

Her father was set against her leaving home. Ann had some heated conversations with him about travel school because he didn't know how trustworthy or accredited they were and would have preferred her to stay in the area and pursue a 'sensible' career. After meeting with a recruiter from the school and more conversations with Ann, he finally relented. She also worked extra jobs and saved money to make it happen.

"I always say that there are two kinds of New Englanders," Ann says, "the ones that grow up here and are happy to drive a few hours and go camping for vacation within the New England states, and the ones who grow up and can't wait to get the heck out. That was me."

Ann did a dozen home-study lessons, then went to Florida for six weeks of full-time training. Her hard work paid off. She was hired right out of school and, at age 19, started her new life in Fort Lauderdale.

After a few years, she moved back to New England and worked as a travel agent. She eventually landed jobs at a succession of large companies doing corporate travel. Ann lived and worked all over the United States. She married and di-

Mary Eisenhauer

"There are two kinds of New Englanders: the ones that grow up here and are happy to... vacation within the New England states, and the ones who grow up and can't wait to get the heck out. That was me."

vorced. "It was a great run," she says. "You either get into travel and you love it and you live, sleep, and breathe travel; or you hate it. I loved it," Ann says. "Even now, I don't like people doing travel reservations for me. I do my own. I thrive on handling the details and making trips happen from beginning to end."

But online travel booking was transforming the industry. While working in the on-site travel office for a Silicon Valley technology company, she had an opportunity to transition to the tech company's education team and jumped at the chance. During her 14-year tenure, her employers provided funding for her college expenses, enabling her to finish her associate and bachelor's degrees; and she enjoyed a second career working in education and corporate alliances.

But even before her transition out of the last company, she knew that change was coming. She was meant to do something different with her life. "I was well on my spiritual path... I had a strong gut feeling of things that were coming. I had taken a number of different personal development classes and done some serious introspection to find out who I was, what I wanted to do, and where I was going in life." She saw that her choice was to either embrace change or let it destroy her. "That's just not who I am," she says. "I would not let the job elimination destroy me. I embrace change."

The path to healing

In the midst of her divorce, Ann moved back to New Hampshire in 2007 and continued to work for the tech company until her position was eliminated in January 2015. She had been volunteering at a local hospital providing Reiki for patients and wanted to do more of that type of work. When she saw a posting for a course to become a licensed nursing assistant, she signed up. She quickly completed the course and immediately found a job at a nursing facility. She loved the residents but eventually found that working for $10 an hour–$11.20 on the night shift–wasn't sustainable. "I think one of the reasons I stayed at the LNA job for as long as I did was because I wanted to help people. But I needed to make a living, too."

In Spring 2021 she took a vacation to the Outer Banks in North Carolina. On the last day of the trip, she went to the Wright Brothers Museum. Ann says the empowering messages on museum posters were exactly what she needed as she began her reinvention. "The messages were jumping out in my face. My creative juices were back again. And I thought, 'I feel energized. I'm going to come back from the past few years with new energy'."

On her way home, she stopped in Virginia Beach for a couple of days to try Edgar Cayce's A.R.E. Health Center & Spa. Ann had massages in the past but never one that connected with her energy the way this one did. She asked the massage therapist where she went to school and was told there was a school on site. Ann went back to her hotel, researched the school, and submitted her application that night.

Mary Eisenhauer

"It's taken a lot of risk, sacrifice, and faith on my part, jumping into the unknown for all of these things."

In October of that same year, Ann moved to Virginia Beach for her training, graduating in 2022 as a licensed massage therapist and finding the missing piece that she had been searching for.

In 2023, she established Ann's ECA Massage in Massachusetts, bringing together her skills in reflexology, medical and relaxation massage, craniosacral therapy, and energy work to create a unique experience for each client based on their individual needs. In her practice, she also does in-home massage medical massage for veterans, satisfying the desire to help as she did when she was a licensed nursing assistant.

She's learning to trust her own voice. "It's taken a lot of risk, sacrifice, and faith on my part, jumping into the unknown for all of these things. I'll continue to take risks to realize my dreams even when family and friends don't see the vision. This life is about service to others and how to give back or pay it forward. It's critical to go with what resonates with you and listen to that inner voice."

Becky McCord

Embrace the Zigzag Path

Becky is a retired military officer who is making a career change to focus on animal care. She lives in Pennsylvania.

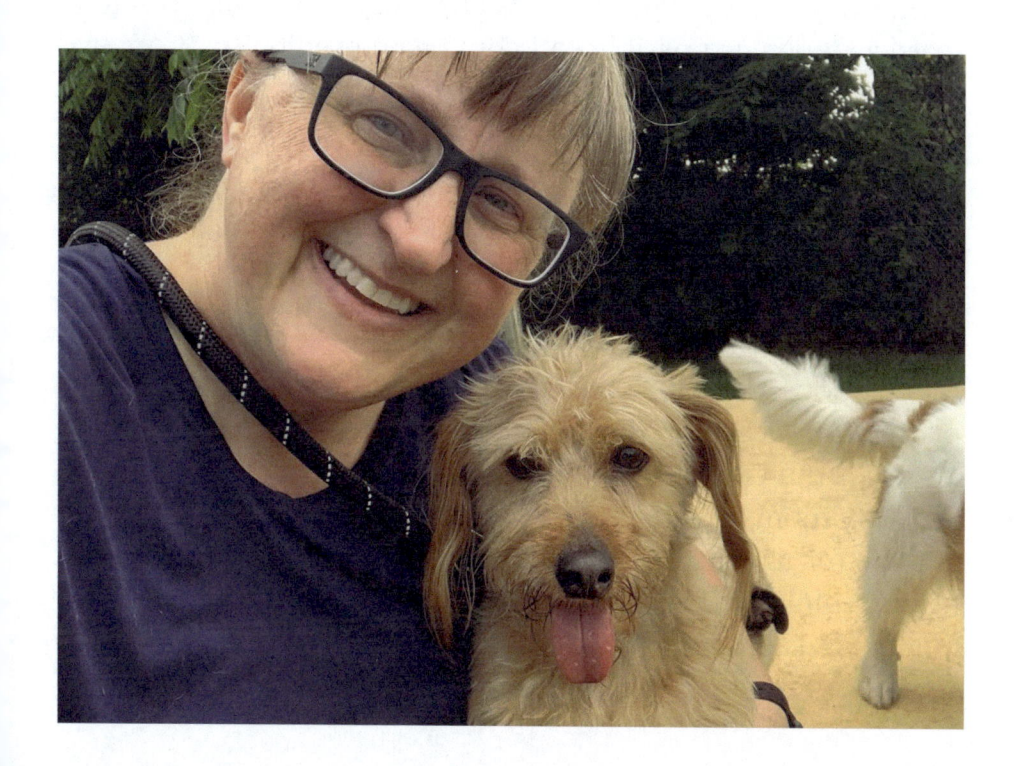

After three decades of active and reserve service in the U.S. military, Becky McCord is back to school, studying biology, ecology, and animal health and behavior. Working in HR is paying the bills, but her heart is in volunteering to work with animals.

Becky was excited and relieved after she decided to retire and enroll in college full-time. "Once I started making those decisions, everything started falling into place, 'like it was meant to be.'"

Becky was only 17 when she first joined the military as an Air Force Academy cadet. After her graduation in 1995, she was assigned as an aircraft maintenance officer at McConnell Air Force Base in Wichita, Kansas. She was one of only three women in a squadron of more than 200 people. She called the experience "eye-opening, it was certainly a unique experience to be one of three women but at the same time, I loved the five years when I was on active duty. I really enjoyed the people I worked with. I enjoyed the work; it was challenging as I was trying to learn as much as possible so I could gain credibility. But it was also stressful in that I was trying to figure out where my role was in all of it."

Role models

Becky remembers the supportive women friends she met during military service, "but I have very few role models, which is sad. I have friends who I look up to for what they do, or how they've done things in their life, or what they've accomplished or who they are, but I don't really have a lot of female role models other than my mom and my grandmother."

"My mom, for sure, is a role model. She raised my brother and me for a while on her own due to a bad first marriage. But I don't think I appreciated how much she had done and how much she sacrificed to take care of my brother and me until she got remarried and had more children. It was clearer to me when I got older just how much she invested in me and in all of my siblings, to make sure we would go on to be educated, productive adults."

Return to service

After her active duty ended, Becky lived in Wichita and joined the Air National Guard unit in Sioux City, Iowa, commuting each month for guard duty.

She was working part-time for a real estate company, recently married, and preparing to go back to school, when she learned about a program that provided alternative certification for veterans to become teachers. Her mother and sister were educators, so it seemed like a good idea and could fit her life well. In 2001, she took a job teaching high-school science in Wichita, Kansas.

But shortly thereafter, she found that teaching wasn't the career for her. She did not feel the same connection to the work or the satisfaction her family members felt as educators. She needed something different.

After 9/11, Becky changed units, joining an Air Force Reserve unit in Wichita. "They said: 'We'd love to have you,'" she says. "I went to school down in Florida for two months, which was great. And then came back and I was on extended active duty, working for different programs that they had in place."

Becky continued to serve in the Air Force Reserve and also worked for the military as a civilian employee, moving between executive support, communications, and aircraft maintenance.

"It gave me some great opportunities to do things that may not have necessarily been in my wheelhouse at the time. I really enjoyed my military career."

Over the years, her expertise in government relations, program management, and command and control took her to posts of increasing responsibility. Becky served in the U.S. Department of State from 2012 to 2017 as a foreign service/general services officer, posted to Athens, Greece.

Retirement

Becky had always planned to remain in the military for 40 years and retire at age 58½. But changes in the military after the COVID-19 pandemic – and changes in her own physical health after she contracted the virus herself – made her recall a conversation with a chief. Back when she was a lieutenant, the chief told her, "You'll know when it's time. And you should leave when you know it's time, because you don't want to be bitter and you don't want to be angry." She knew that the chief meant she should go out on a good note.

Becky retired in July 2022 as a Lieutenant Colonel. Counting her time at the Academy, she had served for 31 years. Her last post was as Chief Future Operations/Battle Watch at the AFRC Force Generation Center at Robins Air Force Base, Georgia.

"I've always tried to leave workplaces better in some way than they were when I started. I don't know that I've always been successful at that, but I like to think that I've made a positive impact in one or two moments."

A zigzag path

"I remember telling my therapist I was going to retire from the military," And she said, 'How are you feeling?' And I said, 'I'm so excited!' I'm thinking about all the opportunities I will have after I retire."

"Like what?" the therapist asked.

"I started talking about how I want to go back and get a degree to work with animals. I'd love to work in a zoo or an aquarium or wildlife sanctuary. This is what I want to do." Becky

> "My entire career has been zigzagging. I've realized that I'm not going to always move in a straight line, And that's okay, that's part of the adventure."

glowed as she explained her interests.

The therapist encouraged her. "She said, 'I can hear the excitement in your voice. I think you're making the right decision.'"

Becky's dream came a step closer when she learned that she was also eligible for retirement from the federal Civil Service. Between that and her veteran's benefits, she found that she was able to go to school full-time. "It was like, once I started making those decisions, everything started falling into place."

Lessons learned

As she returned to civilian life, Becky reflected on her career. "I've learned that I'm not patient at all. I have high expectations of other people," she admits, and says she's learned to "deal with those expectations in a realistic manner because otherwise, I'm going to continue to be disappointed in life.

I also realized that if I put my mind to something, I can do it. But I also have to recognize that I don't always know 100% what I want. And it's OK to try different things and not necessarily stay firmly on one path. That's absolutely what my career was."

She initially applied to a college program for wildlife conservation, but a chance conversation with a woman who worked at an aquarium opened her eyes to that type of work and eventually took Becky in a different direction. "I had to be gracious with myself and say, 'I know this is what you think you want to do, but it isn't.'"

Another zigzag

This course correction is in keeping with the way she's always approached her work life. "My entire career has been zigzagging. I've realized that I'm not going to always move in a straight line, And that's okay, that's part of the adventure. And, although there are days when I just want it to be a straight line, I also know that in the end, when I look back on it like I did with my Air Force and Civil Service career, straight lines aren't always the best way there."

For a while, Becky enjoyed working in a doggy daycare, both for the experience and the extra cash, but she needed to stabilize her time and income so, in late 2023, Becky embraced yet another zigzag when she took a job as a human resources specialist with the Commonwealth of Pennsylvania. "I am really enjoying the HR job, as it is new for me and I'm learning something new every day. Plus, I get to telework three days a week, so that is a great benefit."

Becky plans to start volunteering at a wildlife rescue center once she finishes her degree in animal health and behavior at Unity Environmental University. "It may just be that I have to work with animals in a volunteer capacity for now," she says, but one thing is for sure: Becky McCord will be keeping her eyes out for her next opportunity for reinvention.

Editor's note: Becky checked in just before this book went to press, writing: "I am graduating in September and already looking for somewhere to volunteer!"

You're More Than You Knew

Breaking through: that's the theme of many women who are creating their own midlife reinventions. They are self-aware enough to embrace their failures and grow from the lessons learned. They reach into the past to claim dreams that they once thought were impossible, or confidently set new and exciting goals.

The women in this section have overcome personal setbacks and pushed forward. Each one knows that, after her reinvention, she is so much more than she ever thought possible.

Lorraine Connell

What Kids Need to Hear

Lorraine once spent her days leading a high school chemistry class—but, once she left the classroom, she found her true calling in teaching teens about leading through confidence, resilience, and awareness. Lorraine lives in central New Hampshire.

Lorraine Connell used to teach high school but says that, even though she was changing her curriculum and methods of teaching, there was not a lot of new learning or growth for her.

She was stuck in a hamster-wheel routine, with no time for soul searching to find her real passion: teaching high-school teens about leadership.

As an advisor to a leadership development program

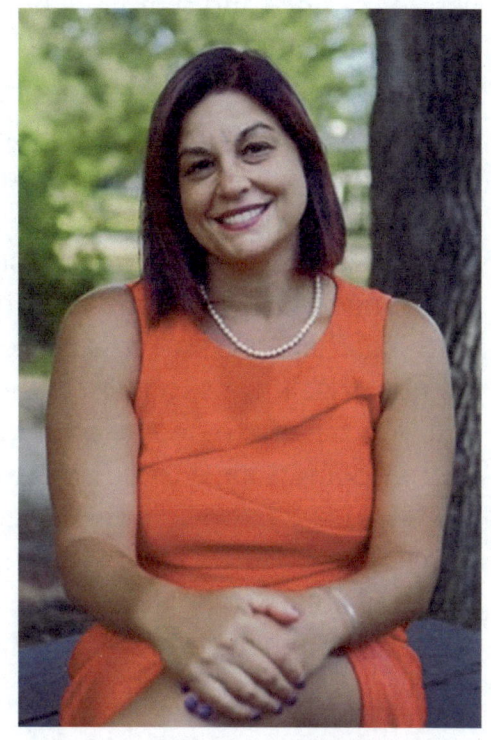

at the public high school where she taught, Lorraine had created a curriculum to help students shape their personal goals and learn teamwork and facilitation skills. She also engaged the community to build connections.

In 2015, after almost 20 years in the classroom, Lorraine left to concentrate full-time on coaching high school students. "I really felt like I could build leadership any place," Lorraine says.

With her husband's income and some substitute teaching to help support her family as she worked on her career change, Lorraine set out to define her new path. She listened to podcasts on how to start a new business and make connections.

Running a business

Once Lorraine stepped away from teaching, her attention turned to coaching. As part of her own career development, she worked with another former teacher who had become a real estate trainer—and that gave her the opportunity to work with real estate agents.

Lorraine developed a course that was approved in two states, but her main focus is still on building connections with parents, college counselors, and coaches to get her message into schools.

She also learning to be a small business owner. "One of the things that I've learned is I have to be really good at a lot of things," she says. "I've said to my husband, I've said to my friends, that I want to just do the thing that I'm really good at, which is talking to people about leadership. But in order to get to that point, I have to be able to market. I have to know what SEO is. I have to be able to do taxes—and, yes, I can farm those things out, but I feel like I'm so small at this point that I don't have the ability to do all of those things."

Lorraine had to redefine what success looked like for her

> "The last myth that we believe about leadership is that you need to be perfect to be a leader. I really try and demystify those beliefs and give kids the authority to see themselves as leaders."

as her start-up began to take root. "One of the biggest obstacles that I have had to face is redefining what success means to me. I have spent the majority of my life measuring success on a salary or on that ladder, moving up for a company or an industry. My first three months in business on my own, I'm defining the success on $600.00 and looking at, 'Oh my gosh, in three months I used to be able to make $15,000'."

Cash flow quickly became an issue. Lorraine realized that a major challenge of focusing her business on teenagers is that her actual client—the student—"doesn't have the means to pay me. I have to convince a stakeholder in that student's life, the principal or the administrator of that school, or the parent of that teen, in a way that doesn't minimize what I'm trying to do."

One problem with that, says Lorraine, is that "schools really believe they are doing leadership." She points out that traditional school programs nurture teens who are already in leadership positions. "What about all the rest of the kids? And what about kids who have applied for a leadership position and didn't get it? What is the message you're sending to those kids? Because I've been that kid and the message to me is that 'Okay, I'm not a leader'—and I don't think that's the message we as schools want to be sending."

What kids need to hear

Lorraine says she's learning to value herself for the work she's doing "in a way that's not tied to a number. From what I've gathered, there are a lot of leadership coaches helping CEOs, but very few are focusing on doing this work with teens."

The result was Peers Not Fears LLC. At the top of the company website is the tagline: "Transforming all students into future leaders." The company works with school administrators, parents, and teens.

Part of Lorraine's job is to teach teens that a lot of their assumptions about leadership are just myths. "In school, we really promote that myth that leadership is a title," Lorraine says. She says that teens make the mistake of thinking, "So if I'm not one of those captains, I'm not a student council president, I guess I'm just not a leader."

Lorraine also debunks the myth that leadership is something you're born with. "There are a lot of us, myself included, that believed that some people have it and some people don't. And if I don't have it, then I don't have it."

"The last myth that we believe about leadership is that you need to be perfect to be a leader," Lorraine says. "I really try and demystify those beliefs and give kids the authority to see themselves as leaders."

Peers not Fears is also home to Lorraine's podcast Today's Leaders: From Teens to Titans, a podcast focused on learning from student voices.

Lessons

Lorraine acknowledges that her new career is a work in progress. "I've learned that a lot of the things that I am trying to do with teens are the same things that I have had to do for myself," she says. "The messages that I am trying to tell students are the same messages that I need to say to myself. And it makes it real for me."

"Just the other day, when I was talking to students about how leadership's not a title, I said, 'How many of you would be comfortable standing up here, doing what I'm doing?' About half of them raised their hand.

"And I said, 'How many of you think that I'm nervous standing up here?' And nobody raised their hand.

"'I'm very nervous,' I said, 'but the message I want to share with you is that people only see what is on the outside, even when we think they can see what's on the inside. It's only you who knows/sees whats happening inside.'"

Lorraine realized that "the message I'm telling them is a message I really need to be still saying to myself. It's kind of neat for me to realize how much learning we all have to do, and should be doing, and will continue to do if we take those risks."

Kendra Hackett

Second and Third Acts, and More

Kendra raised a family and climbed the corporate ladder. At age 52, she turned the satisfaction of her daily gym session into a business that thrived until the COVID-19 pandemic. She's rediscovered her love of performing and writing but found that there was still one more transformation in store for her. Kendra lives in South Carolina.

Kendra Hackett built a decades-long career in corporate human resources, but it was a superhero moment in the gym that changed the path of her own life.

Kendra started her career in talent acquisition right out of college, but after 30 years she felt that the recruiting field had changed. "I was working for a company where people became less important. They were not 'considered people any-

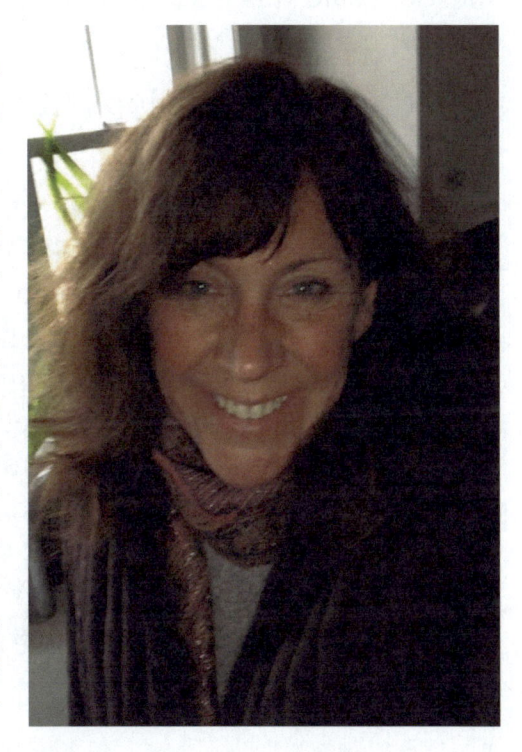

"I recently realized that I have much less fear around change."

more; they were 'talent'. They were just skills, and everything was about numbers. I was merely filling jobs. It wasn't feeding my soul anymore. Helping people find a job and find a better life for themselves was being whitewashed out of the equation."

She was also frustrated that her one-on-one connections within the company were diminished. "Periodically, the management would move recruiters around to support different parts of the business. There didn't seem to be a rhyme or reason. We were just moved. They were taking away my relationships with hiring managers, relationships that were valuable to me. So, I said this isn't working for me. I want to do something else."

What would my life look like?

Her epiphany came from an unlikely place. "I was working out at a gym that I loved," Kendra says. "The workouts were consistently great and I felt like Wonder Woman every time I finished. The concept at this gym was a terrific combination of boxing and weights and cardio and I was seeing great results. I got to know the owner of the gym and we eventually talked about the pros and cons of ownership. I liked the other members of the gym and the camaraderie everyone felt whenever they came in. The feeling there was infectious.

"I worked out at this gym for over a year, and in the middle of a workout one day I thought, 'What would my life look like if I could help other people feel this good?'"

At age 52, Kendra opened her own gym. "I just had this vision of what my life would look like. I envisioned opening several locations of the gym and working with clients to help them realize their fitness goals. Of course, my vision was that it was all going to be lucrative."

Others told her she was crazy. Even her father, who had always told her she could accomplish anything she wanted to, thought she was too old to start a fitness business. "It was discouraging to hear that from people I loved. I just knew that I needed to do something different with my life, after decades of work in the corporate world. I decided to open my own gym anyway." And her midlife reinvention was underway.

Pandemic problems

Soon after she made the decision, Kendra opened the gym. "For the first few years it was wonderful," she says. "I built a clientele of people who gradually became my friends, hired trainers to work for me, and saw clients changing their lives through fitness. It wasn't perfect but it was new and felt great, and offered me the flexibility to be around throughout the day for my high school-aged sons. But then COVID-19 hit. And then it wasn't as wonderful.

"There were glimmers of joy because I was still helping people transform their lives. But as the pandemic was going on, it was a struggle to stay in business. We had no choice but to close for a few months, during which time I tried to continue to engage clients online. That was no small feat. Once the gym reopened, I had a hard time finding and keeping trainers. This meant that I worked long, long hours. Clients of the gym were sometimes afraid to come in, not knowing if they would catch the virus. I spent as much time cleaning as I did working with clients and actually running the business. Some clients became much more cavalier about paying their bills, which of course impacted the gym's bottom line. I could write a whole book of stories of the way people changed. It became exhausting and disheartening.

"The joy quotient was just dropping. The satisfaction I felt when I first opened was gone. As staff turned over, I spent more and more time working; which meant less time with my teenage sons. I spent more and more time chasing clients for their monthly dues, and less time helping clients with their fitness goals. The stress of staying afloat affected my sleeping habits and my overall mindset. COVID changed everything, and I knew I needed to get out for my physical and emotional health. It took time to find a buyer, but I ended up selling the gym."

One more reinvention

Kendra sold, and just months later, her youngest son went to college. "I was looking, not only at what my life would look like without the gym but also at what my life would look like when I was no longer a full-time parent. That reinforced for me that whatever I was going to allow in my life, it needed to be something that sparked joy."

After a couple of months of reflection, she went back to the corporate world, to talent acquisition where she had gotten her start. But this time she found a company more aligned with her values. "I had the opportunity to go back into recruiting with a company that valued all the things that I valued, and a boss that valued her staff as humans and not just as acquirers of talent." It felt right and offered her the financial stability the gym had not. So she accepted the offer.

Kendra soon discovered that there were tradeoffs between entrepreneurship and working for a company. Although she no longer had the freedom of owning her own business, she had control of her time again. "My life had been subsumed by the gym. I slept and I worked, and that was it. There was no time for anything else. On days off, I caught up on sleep and did the minimum to clean my house and pay bills. I barely even saw my kids at the end of my time owning the gym. And I decided that I wanted life in my life. So the pact I made with myself was that I would only do things that brought me joy."

She also regained control of her finances. "As I was making the transition out of entrepreneurship and looking at what I wanted my life to look like, going back into the corporate world was nice because I didn't want to be broke anymore." There was no way she could have anticipated the financial toll that COVID would take on the gym. Going back to the corporate world was the best option. Even better, the job was fully remote, which enabled her to balance work with her outside interests.

Reclaiming an old passion

In the midst of returning to her talent acquisition career, Kendra has built in time to revive some old dreams. Early in life, she had played guitar, and she played French horn in a community band. She loved music but gave it up when her sons were born. Like so many women, she put her interests aside when she became a mother. "I never completely abandoned myself, but my life was work and my children. I don't regret a minute of it."

But after selling the gym, Kendra's creative life came full circle. "One day I was talking to my son, who is living his life, making his dreams come true. And after talking with him I was very sad because I thought What am I doing? He was chasing his dreams. I was returning to Corporate America. But then I got a call from a friend, telling me about a band that was looking for a backup singer. And I thought: 'This could be a lot of fun!'" She debated trying out, having limited singing experience. Although she had performed in choruses, Kendra had mostly sung in the shower and the car. During the pandemic, she had started singing at open mics, as a way to step out of her comfort zone. She found that she loved it.

She joined the band. "It was so much fun being on the stage and singing ...to see people dancing and smiling and enjoying themselves from the perspective of the stage. Just like the open mics, being a backup singer was completely outside of my comfort zone, but I did it." And she spent several months performing at gigs and reliving her love of music.

Since returning to her corporate career, she has also gone back to playing guitar, and has dabbled in theater, taking acting classes and conquering her fear of memorization. "It fed my soul so much so that I actually wrote a one-act play and I'm hoping to have it performed at a play writers' group that I've joined."

Lessons learned

Kendra learned a lot from her time as a business owner. "I learned that I am an excellent motivator, cheerleader, and coach. I love supporting people in the pursuit of their goals and being there to help them keep going when they want to quit. I also learned that I am not a good business person. I don't like chasing people for money. I don't like dealing with bills and creditors and loans, and that was very apparent during the pandemic. During the pandemic, I did rise to find as much assistance as I could for my business. But that was for a defined period of time.

"Going back to the corporate world was a lot easier than I thought it would be. After owning my own business, I am not as concerned with office politics and looking good to my colleagues and being intimidated by people in higher positions than me." I think this has everything to do with my attitude. I know that I am a resource for my colleagues and I have valuable information to share. I am a true partner with managers in the hiring process. It's a very different mindset when you think of yourself as a tool versus a partner."

She now brings her experience as a business owner to the table as a peer. "I have interacted with other business owners, and I have operated at the level that these managers operate at. I know them. I know what they do. I know how they do it."

Kendra also brings a new level of confidence to the job, based on her accomplishments in bringing a business through a global pandemic and coming out on the other side. "My attitude is very different than it was before, and I think that it has a lot to do with my confidence. Those are very powerful lessons that I've taken with me back into the corporate world."

And her experience as a business owner continues to illuminate her re-found corporate career. "I recently realized that I have much less fear around change." I made a quick decision to move from New Hampshire, where I grew up and then raised my boys, to South Carolina. The boys are adults now and I needed a change of scenery after so long in the same place. As I packed up my home, I didn't know exactly where I would be going. I hadn't found a home in South Carolina, so didn't have a definite plan for where I would be living–and it's okay because I know that I can do it. I can do whatever I set my mind to, and that's a lesson that I learned through all of the changes that I've made in my life."

Sue Loncaric

Ageless Attitude

Sue gave up her ballet school for a career in administration management but discovered a midlife passion for running and fitness that led her to create a community and coaching business for Women Living Well After 50. Sue lives in Queensland, Australia.

"I think I've reinvented myself several times throughout my life," says Sue Loncaric. The journey has taken her from a childhood where her dreams were not encouraged to a life of encouraging women around the world.

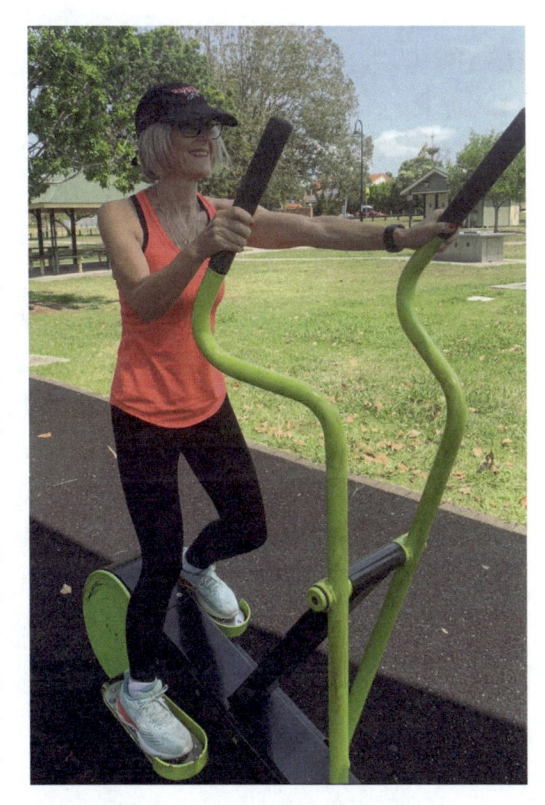

Sue grew up in a working-class family in Sydney, Australia. She attended an all-girls school and went to a very selective high school. A dancer, she started her own ballet school while she was still in high school.

She wanted to be a teacher, but "education for women wasn't really encouraged then," Sue says. Her parents discouraged her, asking, "Why do you want to be a teacher? Why do you want to go to university? You're only going to get married and have children anyway."

"I sort of went along," Sue says. "I just wanted to please them, not doing what I really wanted to do."

Stories and role models

Sue cautions against "those stories that we tell ourselves, going back in time throughout our life when we were told who and what we should be, and what we are capable of; we start to believe that—and in actual fact, it's not that way at all." She says these "limiting beliefs—'Am I good enough?' 'Who do I think I am?' You know, that imposter syndrome: 'Why do I think I could do that?'—stops us from getting out there. That was a big obstacle for me."

Still, Sue says she was inspired by her mother's ability to persevere and the courage with which her mother had faced cancer. "She was such a gentle woman, but she had an inner strength and never complained."

Sue had other role models as well, including an older cousin. "She had such an influence on me because she showed that she could do something with her life. She did have children, but as they got older, she became a librarian. She was always doing short courses and studying to improve herself. She had opinions on politics and all sorts of things, which really impressed me. I always wanted to be like her because she was someone who was starting in her own way to be independent, to be a woman who was living the life that she wanted to live while still being a wife and mother."

Starting over

After a divorce in her 30s, Sue made major changes to her life. She closed her dance school and moved across Australia to another city where she where she worked in financial accounting and business administration for various companies.

She also remarried, creating a blended family with her daughter and son and her husband's two children.

At age 50, encouraged by a group of women who were young enough to be her daughters, she started running. "They had faith in me that I could do it. I'd never run before—I couldn't even run between here and the lamp post—but I built it up and ended up running a half marathon at 50 and then a full marathon at 55."

A few years later, she left the commercial world behind. Her husband, who was a few years older than Sue, was already retired, and they were caring for his elderly parents. Sue wasn't really enjoying her job, so she and her husband agreed that she should take a break. "And so, I took early retirement."

No plan

At 57, Sue found herself without a career for the first time in her life. "I had no plan—and that was my first mistake," she says. "I felt a bit of relief that I was free for the first time in my life... And at first, I thought, 'This is fabulous.' After a few months, I realized that I just wasn't ready for that lifestyle... I needed to find something where I didn't lose my identity. I had been defined by my career, by being a wife, a mother, that sort of thing. I had all these different labels, and now it was a time for me to rediscover who Sue was."

Sue started her midlife reinvention by stepping completely outside her comfort zone to write a blog to connect with other women and build her own self-confidence. "I really wanted to try and encourage women through my experience. I wanted to share what I was going through—to share my stories and my ideas about living healthy."

That blog became her podcast and radio show "Women Living Well After 50." The podcast has run for more than four seasons. "I always ask: 'What does being a woman living well after 50 mean to you?' Sue says. "I've probably done well over 100 interviews and every woman answers differently. And that's what I love. They all have a different take—which is right because it's not just physical exercising or eating well. There are so many ways that we can live well and enrich our life." She says that pushing past her own insecurities (what she calls "the mean girl in my mind") brings her satisfaction. "You feel proud of yourself because you've done something that you never thought you would do."

Sue reinvented herself and her husband worked with a physical trainer, and she realized that she had a passion for becoming a personal trainer and fitness instructor herself. But when she applied for certification, she was told that she was probably too old. "And so I accepted that thought," Sue says. But at age 60, she ran another marathon "and I thought, 'You know what? I'm gonna give this a go.'" She found a mentor and an online course, and with the support of her husband and family, she completed her certification at age 63. Now, she works with women online in a virtual studio for group fitness classes. "I've proved them wrong, but I wasted three or four or five years when I could have been doing something that I really love because I listened to that ageism and self-doubt."

Support system

Sue's husband has been very supportive of her progress, and she also surrounds herself in community. "I think that you need to have cheerleaders around you because sometimes

Mary Eisenhauer

"If people aren't bringing you joy, if what you're doing isn't bringing you joy, you've got to have the courage to let it go."

you're not having a good day and you have a crisis of confidence, and you need someone there to just give you that little 'Yep—Come on, you can do it. We believe in you.'"

She also emphasizes the need to step away from toxic voices. "If people aren't bringing you joy, if what you're doing isn't bringing you joy, you've got to have the courage to let it go. That might be friendships, if someone is not going to be supportive and is trying to hold you back, unfortunately. You may decide to stay friends—but if you do, you don't see that person as often. And if it's really becoming toxic, then you have to learn to have the courage to say, "Well, I'm sorry, I can't have you in my life because you're just not filling me with joy. You're not helping me."

Ageless attitude

On her website, Sue writes: "Let's throw out the word 'age' and replace it with 'ageless'. When we use the word 'age' we immediately throw barriers up or are perceived in a certain way. People may say 'good for your age'—but we shouldn't be defined by that. It is our attitude to life that defines us, not how many years we have been on this planet."

Now, in her 60s, Sue says she has come into her own. "We all have regrets sometimes. But, of course, you can't dwell on that. You have to just say, 'Well, okay, that's how it was'—or, 'That's how I was. And I'm different now. And I'm going to make sure that I do what's right for me.'"

Sue says, "Since I've turned 60, my confidence has increased and I'm doing all these things that people have said, 'Why do you want to do that?' It was a big deal for me to do a podcast when I don't have much self-confidence, but the more you do things that you fear, the more you overcome it."

"I'll have my days where I think, "Who are you?' 'What are you doing this for?' But there are many other days, I feel good—I've just done that, and I feel pretty proud of myself.

"I think I'm proof that you can work on your self-confidence. It's never too late for anything, really."

JoAna McCoy

Completely New and Different

JoAna is ready for a change. After a career in public administration, she reassessed after the COVID-19 pandemic and decided to not just live, but thrive. JoAna lives in North Carolina.

JoAna McCoy grew up in Memphis, Tennessee. "Actually, I'm from the Deep South," she says. "We have the best barbecue going—there's no competition!"

Her life has been grounded in the states of the "Appalachian Triangle," the confluence of Tennessee, Kentucky, and North Carolina. "I attended college in east Tennessee, I lived in central Kentucky, and now I am in central North Carolina," JoAna says.

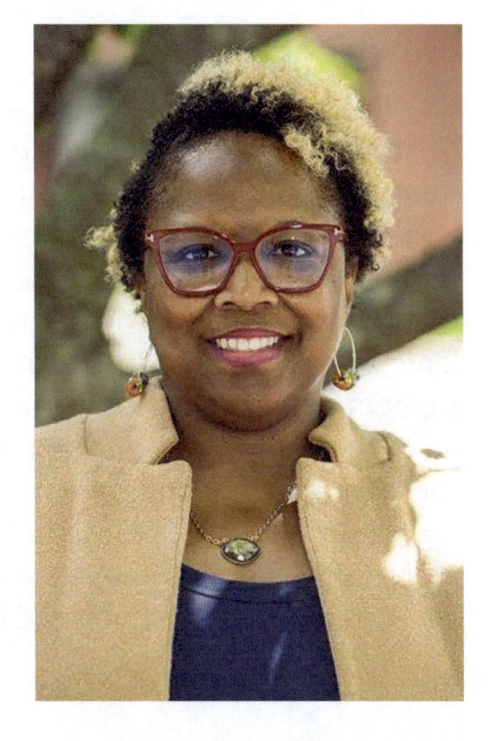

One of JoAna's first college work experiences was in a summer program at Kentucky State University, the oldest of the state's historically black colleges and universities (HBCUs). She says a nighttime dorm supervisor there who became a friend taught her a valuable lesson: "I was particularly frustrated with some of the employees... and one day, she said, 'You just got to meet them where they are and bring them along with you.' That's where I really learned about how our experiences shape us differently."

Her then-husband was a college football coach, so JoAna became what she calls "a trailing spouse—you know, the spouse that's following the spouse with the career. I kind of just took jobs here and there, based upon what was available and what was of interest to me."

Her first jobs were in talent acquisition—a role she hated because "there are so many people that want to talk to you... and everybody gets your phone number. The phone wouldn't stop ringing."

A path to public service

JoAna completed her B.S. at the University of Tennessee at Chattanooga and got her Master of Public Administration from Kentucky State University. Part of her grad-school experience was studying abroad. "It was humbling just to be brought down a whole lot of pegs and notches and realize that I still had a lot to learn and a lot of growth to do. And, that people really were kind; all they wanted in return was kindness. It was really nice to meet genuinely friendly, thoughtful people who didn't have an agenda... And that instilled my thought that there's room at the table for everybody. All of us."

From 2009 to 2013, JoAna worked as Youth Program Director for Kentucky State, then transitioned to a job in the state transportation department's Office for Civil Rights and Small

> "Just because you put the time in, doesn't mean you shouldn't walk away. If at any time it becomes a liability, stop pouring into it."

Business Development, an agency that had funded one of the programs she'd directed at the university. "I wanted to see if theory worked with action," she says. "I met some of the most amazing people I had ever met before in my life," she says. "It was eye-opening and so amazing, and everybody was so warm and so giving. And there I learned how to trust people."

Serendipity

And then, a job offer lured her husband to North Carolina and she JoAna joined the Office of HBCU Outreach in that state's Department of Transportation. "All these little breadcrumbs had been coming together to weave this tapestry. I've worked with students I've worked on the college campus, I've worked in HR, and I've largely directed programs for students and government-funded programs, and that included writing some grants here and there." She'd finished her master's degree in public administration, "and this position open in government was every position I'd had, lumped into one. It just kind of felt like serendipity." She remembers thinking, "I'm completely qualified and I check all the boxes because I've done everything that they're seeking. And the money was right. And I just was like, 'Yes!'"

As program administrator, JoAna's job has been to work with HBCUs and minority-serving institutions to diversify the talent pipeline for Department of Transportation engineering roles, including engineering jobs that have traditionally been dominated by white males. At the time she was hired, only one candidate had been hired out of the program in its nearly 20-year history.

JoAna is proud that more than a dozen people have now been hired through the program. She has created real-world projects and worked with DOT's research center, marketing, and human resources. She's also helped dismantle some of the barriers that candidates faced as they listed HBCU coursework, college credits, and work experience on their resumes—disconnects that she describes as "microaggressions that are frustrating because we're investing in individuals and then we're just throwing the money out the window because we're not trying to retain the talent."

A change in direction

JoAna's oldest child was graduating from high school when the pandemic hit in 2020. She remembers "being at home for a very long time. During that time, I got an opportunity to really sit still and reflect on 'What do I want life to look like?' 'What life can I create?' Because I've always known this was not the final stop. So now, I'm trying to figure out my next step."

Some changes in her personal life prompted other questions, 'because, for the first time in my entire adult life, I'm choosing where I want to live, where I want to do, and what I want, not basing all of those big decisions on someone else's wants. Which is very scary and exciting because this is all completely new and different."

She rejects the idea of staying in a failed job or personal situation just because you've invested time or money in that effort. "Just because you put the time in, doesn't mean you shouldn't walk away. If at any time it becomes a liability, stop pouring into it. It's a sunken cost. Don't keep sinking your money into that."

She has experimented with new interests, from tennis to fostering dogs. The long-term goal turned out to be a desire for a career change into technical project management, which appeals to her sense of order and her preference for tasks with clear start and end dates. JoAna has finished the technical program and has already completed certifications she will need.

Additionally, she is thinking a lot about her personal relationships and talking to her kids about them. "We have real conversations in my household, and I recently was telling them a life lesson that one of the most important career decisions you make is your partner. Your partner makes or breaks your career. Period. A partner helps you determine what choices and chances you take or not take. And your growth because your partner is there to support you."

She's also talked to her children about her life changes. "I think it has helped them understand that you can also change your mind about anything and everything, whenever you get ready."

JoAna continues in her role at the Department of Transportation, but now she's a work in progress. "The good thing is that I get to reinvent me. I get to try something new at this stage in life where I'm full of confidence that I didn't have at 20-something."

Katie O'Leary

What You Manifest

Katie struggled with substance use disorder for many years, but, for the sake of her daughter, she remade her life. Now, she works to help others on their own recovery journey. Katie lives on the south shore of Massachusetts.

Katie O'Leary grew up in a tight-knit Irish Catholic home but lost herself as a young adult in substance use, trying to find her way back to sobriety in the "continuous rat race of doing the same thing that wasn't working for me. I had all of these morals and values, and I kept pushing those lines back to fit my needs."

Katie says she felt broken and depleted, stealing from drug stores to survive.

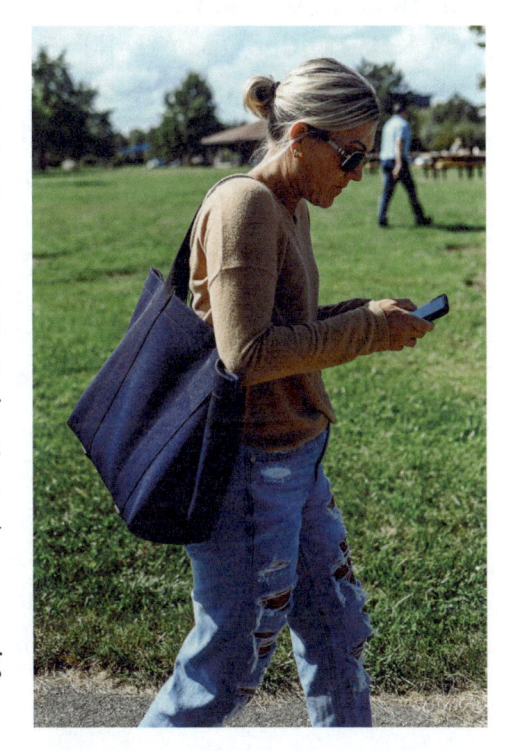

She'd lost custody of her toddler son, and her parents and former in-laws were trying to take her baby daughter. "I was bringing her to places and doing things with her that weren't okay," Katie says now. "She was with me on this really dark journey that no child should ever be present for."

This ends here

The reckoning came when she was fleeing the police after wrecking a stolen rent-a-car. "It was a winter day, maybe 18 inches of snow on the ground, freezing. "I took my little girl and headed outside with her in the cold. We were hiding behind a bush. She didn't even have a jacket on.

"After, like, 30 minutes, she looked at me and was like, 'Mommy, I'm cold.' And in that moment—I don't know, call it God, call it whatever you'd like—but in that moment my heart broke and I knew I was done! I called my dad and asked him to pick us both up so I could once again enter treatment. I knew this needed to end here!"

Katie ended up at HART (Healing and Recovering Together) House, near Boston, and stayed for almost a year. She eventually had both children with her there, and they moved together to transitional housing in her hometown, across the street from her parents.

She held on to her sobriety even when her then-husband relapsed. "I hung on and did what I was supposed to do, and when I went to meetings I raised my hand and just cried and asked for help—and guess what? People helped me."

Recovery

Her ex-husband had a great job but she leaned on him financially while they were married and realized it was time to take care of herself. This is where she came to recognize her own strength. "I found beauty in the struggle. From that pain,

I became a very independent woman. I am very confident and capable that I can not only take care of myself, I can take care of my children. I had so many other goals and aspirations for myself."

Katie has maintained her sobriety for well over a decade. Looking back at her life, Katie says she feels "very blessed to have the experience of addiction because, at the end of the day, it gave me a ton of strength that I didn't know I had. And? It gave me a very distinct voice and empowered me to use it."

Following her own recovery, she started working in recovery services, helping others. "I work in substance use because it's relevant, right, and comfortable, and it's convenient for me." Beginning as a recovery coach,

Katie has built on her own life experiences to create an entire division at North Suffolk Community Services, a large non-profit specializing in behavioral health. "I oversee about 60 people right now as a senior manager. It seems wild to me that this is happening, but I'm dedicated. I love my job."

She also works with courts that deal with people caught up in the criminal justice system and has found that this is the work she is most passionate about.

She has built her own trust network that includes judges and district attorneys. "I've built this rapport with, I would say, powerful people, but to me, they're just humans. I'm learning to keep those boundaries so that I can show up for everybody, so I can show up for myself, most importantly."

Old ambitions, new dreams

As she moves further into midlife, Katie has been revisiting her teenage interests. "I wouldn't say I was weird, but I always kind of gravitated more towards this darker side." She recalls living near a bridge where people sometimes died by suicide, and she was drawn to the scene. "There was always something comforting and peaceful that resonated with me when people transitioned from one life to the next."

She also sought those connections in school. "I started taking biology and anatomy and physiology, just understanding the body and how it worked. And then I wanted to also understand" how does it shut down? How does it break down? What are those components? Where do these diseases come in? I'm more curious about the forensic side."

"I'm not scared of dead people. I want to help people and I feel like I'm extremely empathetic," she says. But her parents didn't understand her interests when she was younger and nudged her "in a very loving way to go to college and explore something else."

That "something else" turned out to be criminal justice classes. "My addiction took off at that point, so I didn't finish school but I was there for three years. I put all of that on the back burner."

"When I got clean and sober, I ended up getting divorced. And in that process, I met somebody else. This person's family just happens to own a funeral home."

Katie says she believes that "what you put out, manifest, comes back to you in some way, shape, or form. And so, this past fall, I started taking classes to become a funeral director."

What specifically draws her to the profession? "The whole process—it's not for the dead person themselves. It's for the living. It's being able to support somebody in that time of need and assist with that grieving process, to make it as safe for the person as possible. I think that's what draws me into it."

She hopes that she and her partner can eventually helm the family business when the time is right. Meanwhile, they share a busy home life with two teenagers and a grade-schooler.

Mary Eisenhauer

"What you put out, manifest, comes back to you in some way, shape, or form."

Saying it out loud

Katie can name many people who have helped and mentored her along the way in big and small ways. "I think honestly, any person I come into contact with teaches me something. It's just a matter of: are you willing to listen?"

That also goes for expressing her feelings for people she cares about. "My parents are wonderful human beings, absolutely wonderful, and they did the best they could with what they had. But what they don't say often is, 'I Love You'; they were never taught how. My mother will write it in a card now, but nobody's ever going to say that. And that's okay. So I make sure that I say that to my kids."

One of the most important lessons she's learned is how to set boundaries for herself. "I am a people-pleaser by nature," Katie says. She says she's learned that "It's okay to say 'No' and I don't owe you an excuse for it. I can just say 'No' because I'm not in a good place, and that's okay."

She's also learned to embrace gratitude. "Gratitude goes a long way, and that's going to change your perception and mindset. The first time I tried to get clean and sober, I went to a therapeutic community and it was like, 'Make a gratitude list and put it in your pocket.' And you know, sometimes I still do that because I can forget really, really, really easy how much work and sacrifice it took, and all of the stuff I had to give up to get to where I am."

Maps for My Own Journey

Developing this book was pure joy: finding midlife women to interview, connecting with them, learning their stories, and realizing how much more alike they are than different.

I knew that every story would be inspiring. I knew that I would meet women with stories vastly different from my own, and that was intriguing. What I did not anticipate was the warm reception I received from each of the women in this book and their common view of the importance of telling these stories. I also continue to be overwhelmed by the enthusiasm my family, friends, and coworkers show for this topic.

Reinvention in midlife sounds daunting, whether done by choice or necessity. Rethinking a career or lifestyle is a privilege, one that requires thoughtful planning and resources. In interviewing these women, I learned that it is financial flexibility, not the size of a person's bank account, that enables bold moves in midlife. Whether finding ways to make extra cash part-time, taking the risk to open a business, trading services with colleagues, or simply taking a leap of faith that plans will work out; these women have adopted flexible financial habits.

These women are also clear in their purpose. In so many different ways, each woman featured in this book recognizes her (sometimes hard-won) privilege and seeks to address unmet needs in her world. Every one of them is making an impact.

And many of these women have overcome adversity in

their lives to get where they are today. Socioeconomic, cultural, interpersonal, and health-related factors have shaped them and ultimately prepared them for reinvention in midlife.

In writing this book, I knew I would be forced to examine my own life choices and entertain my own reinvention. As of this writing, my own midlife bold moves are to be determined, but it is clear that I now have dozens of role models to lead the way.

About the Author

Mary Eisenhauer has spent her career in various roles within Human Resources, and is thrilled to be a first-time author. She is fascinated by human behavior and thoroughly enjoys stories about strong women. She lives in New Hampshire with her husband, two daughters, and two spoiled rescue dogs.

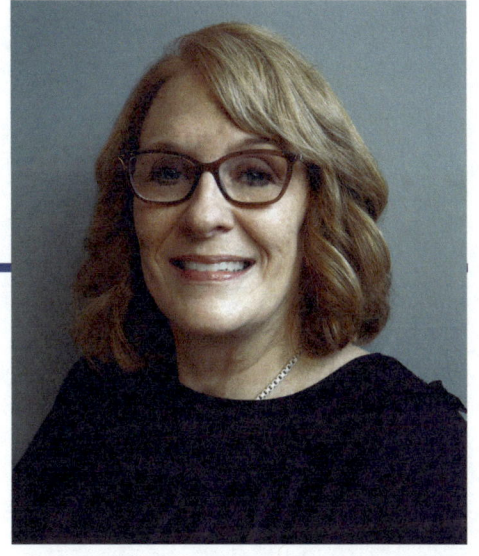

Made in the USA
Columbia, SC
15 January 2025